About the author

Keith Frayn is Emeritus Professor of Human Metabolism in the Oxford Centre for Diabetes, Endocrinology and Metabolism at the University of Oxford. He has spent his career studying human metabolism and nutrition in different conditions, from injured patients in accident and emergency, through studies of exercise and recreational hill-walking, to people with diabetes, obesity and lipid disorders. His recent research has focused on the pathways by which we lay down and mobilise our fat stores.

Keith has published more than 300 scientific articles on nutrition and metabolism, and has been a regular invited and keynote speaker at international conferences on metabolism, obesity, nutrition and cardiovascular disease. His experience in human metabolism is reflected in a number of prestigious awards, including the Sir David Cuthbertson Lecture for the European Society for Parenteral and Enteral Nutrition, the David Murdock Lecture at the Mayo Clinic, the British Nutrition Foundation prize and lecture, and he was the first recipient of the Nutrition Society's Blaxter Award for scientists in the area of whole-body metabolism. He was twice chair of the British Nutrition Foundation's Task Force on Cardiovascular Disease: Diet, Nutrition and Emerging Risk Factors. He is an Honorary Fellow of the Nutrition Society and an Emeritus Fellow of the Royal College of Pathologists.

Other books by the author

Human Metabolism: A Regulatory Perspective (written with Rhys D. Evans, fourth edition, Wiley-Blackwell, 2019)
Understanding Human Metabolism (CUP, 2022)

The Inescapable
Science that Controls
Our Body Weight

A Calorie is a Calorie

KEITH FRAYN

PIATKUS

PIATKUS

First published in Great Britain in 2025 by Piatkus

1 3 5 7 9 10 8 6 4 2

A CIP catalogue record for this book
is available from the British Library.

ISBN 978-0-349-43765-1

Typeset in Sabon by M Rules
Printed and bound in Great Britain by
Clays Ltd, Elcograf S.p.A.

Papers used by Piatkus are from well-managed forests
and other responsible sources.

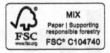

MIX
Paper | Supporting
responsible forestry
FSC® C104740

Piatkus
An imprint of
Little, Brown Book Group
Carmelite House
50 Victoria Embankment
London EC4Y 0DZ

The authorised representative
in the EEA is
Hachette Ireland
8 Castlecourt Centre
Dublin 15, D15 XTP3, Ireland
(email: info@hbgi.ie)

An Hachette UK Company
www.hachette.co.uk

www.littlebrown.co.uk

For Professor John S. Garrow (1929–2016)

Whose common-sense but rigorously scientific approach to the regulation of body weight inspired my own work, and who was a personal guide at a difficult time in my career.

Contents

Introduction

Another book about calories? As I worked on the text for this book, it seemed that every week there would be another article in the newspaper explaining what we should do to lose weight; it felt that every month another book on the topic had appeared. But I found little of that expanding literature satisfying. I am an experimental scientist. I worked in the field of hormones and metabolism for nearly fifty years. I know what the science tells us about insulin, for example, and its role in fat storage – indeed, I think I can say that I have contributed significantly to that literature. But I see half-truths and pseudo-science being peddled. How, then, is the reader to know what to believe or not to believe?

In particular, recent years have seen increasing challenges to the old belief that we have to balance our calories in and our calories out. If we don't, we can expect our weight to change. But, people have argued, if it were that simple, why is it that telling people to eat less and exercise more doesn't seem to help? And isn't the real problem that, while some of us might be blessed with a super-fast metabolism to burn off the excess, most people struggle the other way? I don't think many people (scientists included) realise just how readily we make snapshot judgements of people's metabolism, often based on very shaky evidence. But there is a lot of science showing just how easily we are misled.

I wanted to set the record straight: the record, as I see it, based on my long career in human metabolism. I am not going to add to the plethora of books telling you what, or what not, to eat. In any case, what we eat is only one side of the story: the balance between calories in and calories out. Far less has been written about the 'calories out' side, and yet the two are intimately linked and need to be viewed as a whole. This book will present the science behind 'calories in–calories out'. In later chapters I shall tell you what we know from decades of research about what people eat and how much they exercise, and their effects on body weight. An understanding of the science of energy balance has to underpin anyone's attempts to regulate their own body weight.

My specific research interests for the past few decades have been in understanding how the body handles the nutrients that we eat, how they interact, and how we store them away and then release them from stores when needed. I have, for the last half of my career, worked especially on the way in which our bodies store and mobilise fat. Those interests led, naturally, to my assimilation into the obesity and diabetes research fields, and acquaintance with many of the senior and influential figures in that field.

My own research has covered a number of clinical aspects. For a large part of my early career, I worked in a research unit established by the UK Medical Research Council, the MRC Trauma Unit, based in Manchester, with a remit to investigate the metabolic changes in people who had been injured, or were otherwise seriously ill. That led me gradually into the question of how best to feed such patients to aid their recovery. About mid-career, I moved to a diabetes research unit at the University of Oxford, which gave me the opportunity to study not just people with diabetes, obesity and other metabolic issues but also broader questions about how nutrients interact within the body. From this long and varied experience in human metabolism, I have developed views about how the human body works. My experience of studying what would be called 'intermediary metabolism' – what goes on inside our bodies – has given me very clear opinions on the energy balance and body weight issue. Anyone who knows me will recognise it when I say that I am a firm believer in the idea that energy balance underlies human body weight regulation. I often summarise this as 'it all comes down to calories in–calories out'. I do not believe we need to invent alternative ways of looking at the issue. But more and more I find that I am out on a limb in this belief. That is what spurred me to write this book.

I know that what I have to say will be controversial. I will present my view of the science that underlies body weight regulation. Others have different views, and many have put these in writing. I certainly don't want to offend anyone who thinks that I am making light of the difficulties in regulating one's body weight. Indeed, I shall try very hard to explain exactly why I think this is extraordinarily difficult – as witnessed by the growing tide of obesity despite lots of public-health advice. Certainly, I agree, it's not helping the situation to advise people to eat less and exercise more. But I don't think that advice is unsound: I just think it's inadequate in today's world. I shall explain how I think the environment in the developed world would have to change to make such behavioural alterations more realistic. Lastly, I am not in any way trying to be critical of those who have issues with body weight. I understand those issues. There are sound reasons for them. 'Fat-shaming' is neither useful nor appropriate. And for those who are comfortable with body sizes that others might think inappropriate, I have no argument at an individual level – although the public-health implications of large numbers of people with elevated body weights are clear.

I am a scientist and a science writer. This is a science book, but one that I hope will help the reader in seeing what's important in relation to body weight. I have tried very hard to make it readable by anyone. My experience with my last book, *Understanding Human Metabolism*, has shown me that I must not make assumptions about the readership's background in science. I hope I have produced something that will be readable, interesting and informative.

1

Human energy balance: A concept under threat

The world is getting rapidly fatter. In the twenty-four hours before you read this, the human race will have accumulated an additional 1,000 tons of fat. And with that comes a tide of diabetes, heart disease, cancer and other diseases. Covid-19 arrived at the beginning of 2020. By the middle of 2022, most governments had accepted that this threat has now been managed through a combination of public-health messages and medical developments. Yet, despite decades of public-health advice to eat less and exercise more, and millions of dollars of investment by the pharmaceutical industry, and billions spent on obesity-related healthcare, we seem unable to stem the advance of obesity, even though the underlying cause seems so clear.

No surprise, then, that many people, experts in the field included, have begun to question whether we have the correct understanding of the forces that shape our body weight. Everyday experience also suggests that things are not as simple as the old message of 'calories in–calories out'. We all know someone who doesn't seem to obey the same rules – someone who can eat whatever they like and still not gain weight, or, conversely, someone who struggles to maintain a constant weight while apparently eating almost nothing.

Here's how the counter-arguments go. A pair of scales has 'calories in' on one side, 'calories out' on the other, together with a block of colour representing 'weight gain'. 'Now, who here believes that?' asks the American paediatrician Robert Lustig in a YouTube video viewed more than twenty million times. His audience chuckle apprehensively, sensing that their simple views are about to be challenged. 'I used to believe that,' says Lustig, 'I don't any more. I think that is the biggest mistake. And that is the phenomenon I'm going to try to debunk.'[1]

The concept of 'calories in–calories out', more properly called 'the energy balance model', asserts that if we take in more energy than we expend, we will store the rest. Conversely, if we expend more than we take in, our energy stores will be depleted, and hence our weight will fall. It underpins all public-health advice about maintaining a healthy body weight. But now it is under unprecedented challenge.

Our daily experiences all seem to point to the fact that we just do not understand what makes some people put on weight easily, while others stay lean apparently without effort. Is it possible that some people have a naturally 'fast metabolism' whereas others are stuck with an inability to burn off excess calories? Or could it be, as more and more people are arguing, experts in the field included, that our understanding of human energy balance is flawed, that there are different forces at work, and that we need to rethink our approaches to body weight – and that alternatives to the energy balance model are needed?

I have just been out for a run with my jogging friends Alex

and Bobby.* Alex is large framed, tall and muscular, and does a lot of weight training; Bobby is tiny in all ways, 'petite' one would say. We talked about whether we eat before jogging. One of my companions, it transpires, never eats before jogging, then will come home and have some porridge, then nothing more before an evening meal and bed. The other likes cereals and fruit before jogging, toast afterwards, then a succession of meals, it seems, throughout the day. Needless to say, it's Bobby, the petite one, who seems to eat continuously, Alex who hardly seems to eat at all.

I am sure this sort of conversation is familiar to most people. Indeed, the idea that some people can eat as much as they want but not put on weight, whereas others only have to look at a cream bun to find their waistline expanding, is entrenched even in the professional literature. In 2019 scientists from Cambridge conducted a genetic study of thin people. The accompanying press release on the University of Cambridge website states: 'We already know that people can be thin for different reasons. Some people are just not that interested in food *whereas others can eat what they like, but never put on weight*' (my italics).[2] The prestigious Harvard Medical School has on its website the question:

> Everyone knows some people *who can eat ice cream, cake, and whatever else they want and still not gain weight. At the other extreme are people who seem to gain weight no matter how little they eat.* Why? What are the causes of obesity? What allows one person *to remain thin without effort* but demands that another struggle to avoid gaining weight or regaining the pounds he or she has lost previously?[3] (My italics.)

---

* I have changed the names.

The late well-respected obesity researcher and physician John Garrow, Professor of Human Nutrition in London, whose work we shall discuss many times, dedicated the first edition of his book *Energy Balance and Obesity in Man* to his wife Katharine with the words: 'To K.J.G., 1.72 m, 62 kg, who eats what she likes'. That's someone else with an extra-fast metabolism, then? As we shall see later, John Garrow was an acute observer of eating habits, including his own.

What does 'energy balance' mean?

The eighteenth-century French chemist Antoine Lavoisier, who first named oxygen, was interested in the processes that go on inside our bodies. He showed that we take oxygen from the air that we breathe in, and use that oxygen to 'burn' foodstuffs, in the process liberating energy. I put 'burn' in inverted commas. Foodstuffs do not burn with flames within our cells. They are broken down and combined with oxygen in a series of small steps (each a chemical reaction). The technical term for this is 'oxidation'. But what Lavoisier showed is that the end-result is the same as if they had been burned in a flame. He concluded '*La respiration est donc une combustion*'[4]– respiration is a form of combustion. He used the term 'respiration' here to mean, not the act of breathing but the processes within our bodies (in fact, within our cells) that bring about oxidation of nutrients.

Lavoisier saw that the energy derived from oxidation of nutrients is liberated from the body as heat – just as when substances are burned. He did not have the means to measure heat output from the human body. But he and his contemporaries, including Adair Crawford in Edinburgh, did that with small mammals such as mice and guinea pigs.[5] Lavoisier put them in an insulated chamber surrounded by ice, in turn surrounded by another packed with snow – which acted as an insulator – and measured the heat produced by seeing how much of the ice melted.[6] But he was able to study human metabolism in another way, by studying his assistant, Armand Séguin, using a mask to collect the air that Séguin breathed out. Lavoisier showed that Séguin used more oxygen when he was digesting a meal, or exercising, or subjected to a cold environment. When foodstuffs (carbohydrates, fats and proteins) are oxidised, the products are heat, water and carbon dioxide. (Proteins also contain nitrogen, which is converted into other things in the body, mainly the compound urea.) We breathe out the carbon dioxide. Lavoisier measured the amount of carbon dioxide that Séguin breathed out and showed that it corresponded with the amount of oxygen used – it was another aspect of 'combustion'.

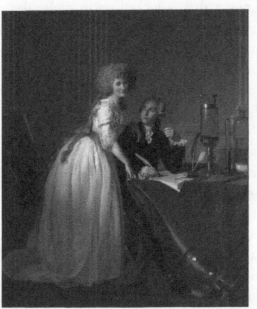

Credit: Metropolitan Museum of Art, New York

Antoine and Marie Anne Lavoisier, by Jacques Louis David (1788). I note that neither appears to struggle with weight issues. In later chapters we will look at what has changed in the intervening 250 years.

Lavoisier could not perform longer-term experiments. An engraving from the time, based on a drawing made by Madame Lavoisier, shows poor Séguin with an uncomfortable-looking copper mask over his face, connected by rigid pipes to a large flask in which the expired air was collected; clearly, he would not have been able to carry that around with him. But Lavoisier would surely have understood that if Séguin had taken in more food than his body could oxidise, then the excess would have been stored in his body. Alternatively, had Séguin eaten less than was required to perform the exercise that he was asked to do, then his body would have needed to draw upon some form of energy stored within it. Those two ideas take us to the heart of human energy balance.

We cannot easily measure the 'energy' stored in the human body. And anyway, what does this mean? When we talk about energy balance, we are referring to chemical energy. Chemical energy is energy that is locked up in molecules and can be released, usually when the molecule is broken apart, as it is in oxidation. When this oxidation occurs within our cells, as I mentioned before, it takes place in a series of small steps. But, ultimately, the energy liberated is exactly the same as if the material had simply been burned. (That was Lavoisier's insight.) Within our cells, some of this energy will be captured for processes within the cell; for example, if it is a muscle cell, for contraction of the muscle; if it is a nerve cell, for moving charged atoms (ions) across the cell membrane to conduct a signal to an adjacent cell. Some will also be lost directly as heat. Ultimately, it will all be lost as heat, but this 'ultimately' might be a long way ahead: suppose, for example, that the energy is used to create more molecules of something different (like building up proteins), the heat will not be lost until eventually that new component is itself broken down.

There is a fundamental law in physics, the First Law of Thermodynamics, sometimes called the Law of Conservation of Energy, that states that energy can neither be created nor destroyed: in any isolated system, the total amount of energy is constant, although it might be interconverted between different forms of energy; for example, chemical energy may be converted to heat. It is clearly simplistic to attempt to apply that to the human body, which is far from an isolated system: things (food and excreta, for example) are entering and leaving the body, and heat is being lost to the environment. But an application of the principle in the broadest terms would indicate that chemical energy taken in (as food or drink) and energy lost as heat, or as some form of work, or excreted, must balance unless there is a change in the internal energy of the body. In turn, the internal energy of the body can mean many things. In the short term, after a meal for example, it might mean a change in body temperature; but body temperature is relatively stable over long periods, and then it's difficult to see what a change in internal energy would mean other than a change in the body's fuel stores. And our main fuel store is fat, as we shall see during the next few chapters.

This is one way of looking at energy balance. We can say that if somebody's weight is stable, on average they must be expending as much energy as they are consuming in food. Strictly, we must say 'as they are extracting from their food', as there is always the possibility that not all the food eaten is used by the body, and that this might vary from person to person. And, when we consider 'energy expenditure', we must recognise that it may take many forms – not just physical activity, but also heat released from metabolism, even during sleep. Alternatively, if someone is gaining or losing weight, we can say that there must be a difference between the energy that they are obtaining from food and the energy they are expending. These concepts have been understood for centuries. The school of animal scientists, working especially in France and Germany in the nineteenth century, investigated the nutritional requirements of farm animals by feeding them different diets and noting the changes in growth and in what was excreted. Detailed human energy balance studies, as we shall see in the next chapter, were first conducted more than 100 years ago.

Although there are challenges now to the energy balance model, I am far from alone in saying that we must continue to believe in it. Jim Hill, Professor and Head of the Department of Nutrition Sciences at the University of Alabama at Birmingham, and Director of the UAB Nutrition Obesity Research Center, has served as president of both the American Society for Nutrition and the Obesity Society. He is a co-founder of the National Weight Control Registry (NWCR), said to be the largest prospective investigation of long-term successful weight loss maintenance: it is tracking over 10,000 individuals who have lost significant amounts of weight and kept it off for long periods of time.[7] (We shall look at data from that study in later chapters.) Hill has written authoritative papers on human energy balance, and describes how 'an understanding of energy balance can help develop strategies to reduce obesity'.[8] When I spoke to him while preparing this text, he said he was very pleased that I was writing such a book. (Jim Hill and his colleague Holly Wyatt have written their own version, *State of Slim*, based on their experiences in Colorado, which has the lowest obesity rate of all the American states.) But others have pointed out the difficulties with the concept of energy balance. The late J.P. Flatt, of the University of Massachusetts Medical School, wrote about these issues since the 1960s and is regarded as something of a grandfather figure in the field. In a thoughtful review article published in 2011, entitled 'Issues and misconceptions about obesity', he discussed why the concept of energy balance can lead to misunderstandings,[9] mainly because we should not assume that the body is in any way trying to maintain a balance of 'energy in' and 'energy out'. Perhaps, he suggested, that is one reason why the energy balance concept is increasingly questioned by many in the field, as we shall now examine.

Perceived problems with the idea of energy balance

Challenges to the energy balance model for understanding human body weight have been around for several decades. But over the past few years they have grown in intensity – together with the scientific weight behind those challenges.

Why should the energy balance model be challenged? Well, firstly, our common perceptions challenge it. Alex and Bobby, my jogging friends, exemplify this. We all tend to make judgements about other people's behaviour based on very flimsy evidence. Here's another personal example. My colleague Fredrik Karpe, who runs the Oxford BioBank and provided data that I have used in some of the chapters, joined our research group many years ago from Sweden. Fredrik, like most Swedes, enjoys the outdoor life, and for several years persuaded me and another colleague to join him on a cross-country skiing tour in the remote Swedish mountains. One year, heavy snow prevented us from getting to our intended starting point, so we put up for a night in a nearby hotel. In the evening they served a buffet of Scandinavian food. Since working in a laboratory in Sweden in the early 1990s, I have had a great liking for the Scandinavian way of life, and indeed for Scandinavian food, so I was, of course, tempted at the buffet to a second, and probably a third, helping, trying the different dishes on offer. Fredrik remarked somewhat scornfully, 'You eat such a lot more than me, Keith. You must have a very fast metabolism.' Yes, Fredrik, I do when we are on holiday, there is a tempting buffet of food that I can't normally eat, and we are about to spend several days skiing in the wilderness. But I don't usually. And actually, because my 'metabolism' has been measured on many occasions, I know that there's nothing exceptional about it. Fredrik and I are, respectively, Professor of Metabolic Medicine and Emeritus (retired) Professor of Human Metabolism at the University of Oxford. Even supposedly well-informed people can jump to erroneous conclusions from snapshots of eating behaviour.*

A more serious consideration, though, is that obesity continues to increase while we seem to be doing the right things to stop it. The US Centers for Disease Control and Prevention (CDC) survey, the National Health and Nutrition Examination Survey (NHANES), reports annually on nutrient and energy consumption by a representative sample of the US population. Their data for males aged 20+ for 2001/2 show a daily intake of 2,620 kcal; for females the figure is 1,850 kcal.[10] The equivalent data for 2017/18[11] show figures of 2,490 kcal and 1,850 kcal respectively: energy consumption by men appeared to fall by 5 per cent, while that of women remained unchanged. Over an approximately similar period, data from the US National Health Interview Survey, covering the years 1997–2017, show a steady increase in the percentage of adults who met physical activity guidelines for leisure-time aerobic activity.[12] (The data are based on household interviews.) And yet the prevalence of obesity continues to increase. Again, the CDC provide the data for US citizens: 'from 1999–2000 through 2017/18, US obesity prevalence increased from 31 per cent to 42 per cent. During the same time, the prevalence of severe obesity increased from 5 per cent to 9 per cent.'[13]

In the United Kingdom, figures are similar. Public Health England, a branch of the UK government, conducts an

---

* Fredrik would like me to say that he now knows better.

annual survey of household and individual food and nutrient consumption. Summary data for a recent eleven-year period, 2008–2019, show a steady decline in energy intake in all age groups and both sexes.[14] The UK's Active Lives Survey by Sport England, an 'arms-length body of government', gives data on physical activity in the population. It covers a more limited time span, but nevertheless over the years 2015/16 to 2019/20 the percentage of those surveyed (almost 200,000 individuals) who met the criteria for being 'physically active' was fairly constant.[15] But, yet again, the proportion of the adult population who are overweight or obese has continued to climb over these periods. The National Health Service (NHS) Health Survey for England shows that the proportion of English men classified as 'obese or overweight' increased from 58 per cent to 68 per cent over the period 1993–2019; for women, the increase was from 49 per cent to 60 per cent.[16]

Very recent global data show the changes from 1990 to 2022. The worldwide prevalence of being underweight has fallen, while the prevalence of obesity has increased dramatically in many countries, including in children.[17] And yet it is difficult to believe that the public-health messages about weight have not percolated through to practically everyone.

What are we to think? Perhaps all our attention, which has been focused on encouraging people to eat less and exercise more, has been misplaced. This is the starting point for much of the current debate.

A good flavour of the recent discussion among nutritional scientists is given by a 'Perspective' article published in 2021 in the *American Journal of Clinical Nutrition*, a flagship journal of the American Society of Nutrition, by David Ludwig, endocrinologist and researcher at Boston Children's Hospital and Professor of Pediatrics at Harvard Medical School, together with a group of seventeen international and well-respected authorities in this field as co-authors. This, therefore, is a powerful and persuasive group arguing against what I myself have come to believe after a long career in metabolism. The thrust of their argument is this. The epidemic of obesity in developed countries continues apparently without pause. Our attempts to counter this epidemic have centred on the issue of energy imbalance. And yet, to quote the authors, 'obesity rates remain at historic highs, despite a persistent focus on eating less and moving more, as guided by the energy balance model (EBM). This public-health failure may arise from a fundamental limitation of the EBM itself.'[18]

These eminent authors instead suggest a model in which carbohydrate intake plays the dominant role, acting through the hormone insulin: 'in the carbohydrate-insulin model (CIM), a crucial effect of diet is metabolic, by influencing substrate partitioning. Rapidly digestible carbohydrates, acting through insulin and other hormones, cause increased fat deposition, and thereby drive a positive energy balance.' This carbohydrate-insulin model has been widely promoted in recent years as the key to understanding human body-weight issues. The American science journalist Gary Taubes has been one of its major champions. (Taubes is a co-author on the paper by David Ludwig mentioned above.) Indeed, in a direct challenge to the medical establishment, Taubes published an essay in the *British Medical Journal* in 2013 in which he argued, as he has in his books, that 'the wrong hypothesis [the energy balance model] won out and that it is this hypothesis, along with substandard science, that has exacerbated the obesity crisis and the related chronic diseases'.[19] The energy balance model is not just wrong, he implies, but it is actually making obesity worse.

An emphasis on carbohydrate intake and its metabolic effects has been a consistent theme in challenges to the energy balance model. If this were the case, changes in carbohydrate intake would be the key to solving the obesity issue. And, undoubtedly, for many people a reduction in carbohydrate intake does seem to have been helpful in managing body weight. So is it time to abandon the concept of energy balance and focus instead upon individual nutrients, especially carbo-hydrates, in the diet?

But there are other, and sometimes opposite, views of the roles of individual nutrients. J.P. Flatt, in the article mentioned earlier, states that 'it is not surprising that a high incidence of obesity is typically encountered in sedentary populations consuming diets providing substantial amounts of fat ... In most animal models high-fat diets similarly promote fat accumulation.' Perhaps, then, we ought to be thinking about fat in the same way as carbohydrate. But I would say that any focus on individual nutrients distracts us from the centrality of energy balance. I will argue in later chapters that metabolic effects of individual nutrients, how-ever much they might seem related to energy storage and release, cannot in themselves cause changes in body weight: a calorie is a calorie, whether it be from carbohydrate or fat or protein. And the key issue is that if our weight is on an upward (or downward) trajectory and we want to change that situation, we need to adjust the balance between 'calories in' and 'calories out'.

A recent development is the idea that something in our environment has changed – other than the rather obvious availability of attractive, energy-rich foods and a panoply of labour-saving devices. Again, a serious body of academics, led by Robert Lustig, has been putting forward the idea that some chemical contaminant in the environment is changing the way we store excess energy: the 'obesogen hypothesis'.[20] That bears some similarity to the idea, popular a decade or two ago but now out of favour, of a viral cause of obesity.[21] I wouldn't argue that either of these cannot be true. But I would argue strongly that they are quite unnecessary hypotheses, and that science mostly progresses by taking the simplest explanation for observations. I think we all know what that is.

I receive a steady stream of emails from people who have read my student textbook on human metabolism, sometimes commenting what hard going it was (it was never intended for the general public), but contacting me because they think I will be able to shed light on their difficulties with body weight, or else that I will support their latest ideas on how to deal with weight issues – or even run marathons. Here's a recent example from Chris, a regular correspondent. 'Would a period of time restricted eating (fasting until lunch) paired with controlled dietary fat intake during the feeding window result in a net fat loss if the total daily kcal consumption equals or exceed the kcals expended?' I'm afraid that my response was once again that it all comes down to calories in–calories out. Time-restricted eating, intermittent fasting – so many of these ideas are just ways of altering energy intake: they do not change the underlying principle of energy balance.

My own belief, which I shall set out over the coming chapters, is that we – even the experts – are easily misled over questions of energy balance. Our knowledge is based upon shaky observations. And even if intake of individual nutrients can be manipulated to give short-term effects, that is a feature of energy balance, calories in versus calories out, not of special metabolic effects of individual nutrients, as many believe.

Issues closely related with body-weight regulation

When I happen to mention that my career has been spent studying human metabolism, it never fails to attract a response such as 'Oh, can you tell me why mine is so slow?' As we have seen, there is a persistent belief that some people (usually other people) just have an innate ability to 'burn off' excess calories – to 'eat ice cream, cake, and whatever else they want and still not gain weight', as the Harvard Medical School sees it. Indeed, since I have somehow remained slim for most of my life, I must admit that I have also sometimes wondered if I have such a 'trick' of metabolism. Certainly, the question has been asked of me many times when I have given lectures on obesity or how we store fat in our bodies, 'What can you know about it, Keith?' And, in writing about obesity, I know that the criticism may be levelled against me that I do not seem to have had the same struggles with body weight that others have. But – as a professional, academic scientist – what I can offer is, I hope, an objective, science-based view of all the issues.

Such major differences, as they must be, in the ability to 'burn off' nutrients, do not directly contradict the idea of energy balance. These fast metabolisers, and likewise the unfortunate slow metabolisers, are not violating any physical principle. And yet, if these differences between people really do exist, they make any generalisations impossible. Perhaps the energy balance model fails because we expect everyone to behave the same (in a metabolic sense), whereas in fact there are wide differences between us. In a similar way, there is increasing realisation that we do not all respond in the same way to medicines, and a large, randomised placebo-controlled study, once seen as the bedrock of modern evidence-based medical practice, may fail because of intrinsic differences in how people respond to the same treatment.[22] Perhaps, instead of a public-health message aimed at increasing physical activity and decreasing energy intake, we need instead a much more individualised approach. While, as I say, differences in 'metabolic speed' (if they do indeed exist to the extent that many believe) do not directly contradict the energy balance model, they do render it considerably less useful than we might hope, and perhaps they might contribute to its apparent failure. *Whether* these differences exist to the extent that we all seem to believe is material for later consideration.

There is another closely related issue: the term 'healthy eating'. It's a phrase I often use myself without necessarily thinking through exactly what I mean. There is no doubt that what we eat can profoundly affect our health in many ways. Our diet affects our risks of serious diseases such as heart attacks and strokes as well as some cancers. Some of these effects may be related to our body weight, but there are also effects that are independent of any change in body weight. We might define a 'healthy diet' as one that is optimal for our long-term health. That would include a diet that helps to control our body weight, since being overweight increases the risks of many diseases (type-2 diabetes as well as those mentioned just now), but it might also refer to other aspects. An example is the type of fat we eat. Nutritionists are almost unanimous in saying we should limit our consumption of saturated fats (the harder fats that come mainly from animal products). Saturated fats can raise the level of cholesterol in the blood, which is closely related to the risk of heart attack and stroke.* But, I will argue in a later chapter, we should not confuse this with the effects on body weight. There is no good evidence that one type of fat (saturated or unsaturated) has a greater effect on body weight than another: they contain almost equal calories, and that's what our body weight depends upon. Of course, if reduction of some nutrient were to improve both energy balance and risk of diseases, that would be a benefit – it would certainly qualify as 'healthy eating': but it is not necessarily so. I shall try to distinguish these effects, without diminishing the importance of either.

---

* This idea has recently been challenged, and it may be that some saturated fatty acids are more harmful in this respect than others. But there are other adverse effects of saturated fat that still lead authoritative bodies to recommend that we limit their consumption.

To illustrate this, I have looked at the latest evidence on what diet we should be eating for health – reducing cardiovascular disease, diabetes, cancer and other non-communicable diseases. The summary from multiple sources is clear that 'healthier alternatives are higher in plant-based foods, including fresh fruits and vegetables, whole grains, legumes [peas, beans and lentils], seeds, and nuts, and lower in animal-based foods, particularly fatty and processed meats'.[23] In a large study of the UK population, dietary patterns that were high in sugar-sweetened drinks, fruit juice, butter and with a high energy content, and low in fruit and vegetable intake, were associated with the greatest risk of cardiovascular disease.[24] (It's funny to think that advice has not really changed over the several decades that I have been in nutritional research.) As the British Nutrition Foundation advises, 'We probably know that we should not have too many foods or drinks that are high in saturated fat, salt and sugar such as chocolate, cakes, biscuits, pastry, crisps and fried chips.'[25] It's striking, as we will see in the course of our look at energy balance, that a diet good for metabolic health is practically the same as one that will help you balance the calories in and out.

To come back, then, to 'a calorie is a calorie': something I have said many times when asked about various ideas that would seem to dodge the whole concept of energy balance. I find it disturbing that there are so many challenges nowadays to this model, with its 250-year history. My concern is that these challenges are distracting us from attention to the real issue: if we are to contain the present epidemic of obesity, we need to find ways that make it possible for people to take in less energy and expend more. There is no alternative, unpalatable though that thought might be. We shall spend the next few chapters looking at just why it's so easy to challenge the energy balance model – and also, why I think those challenges are misplaced.

Units of Energy

As you have gathered by now, this book is about energy so before we go into detail in the following chapters, let me explain. Calories are a unit to measure energy. Scientists now mostly use a different unit, joules, but in nutrition, calories are so widespread that I decided to use them in this book. (And anyway 'A joule is a joule' just doesn't have the same ring for a book title.)

One calorie was originally defined as the heat needed to raise the temperature of one gram of water by one degree Celsius. That's a very small amount of heat. If you boil half a litre of water in your kettle, you will need to put in about 40,000 calories, so we usually work in units of 1,000 calories. At one time these were confusingly called 'Calories'. I will call them 'kilocalories', abbreviated kcal (1 kcal = 1,000 calories). The average human loses about 2,500 kcal of heat per day. (As we will learn, we also take in a similar amount of energy in food.)

Scientists now define 1 calorie as 4.18 joules, since the joule is a more fundamental unit. (It's abbreviated J.) Then our daily loss of 2,500 kilocalories is around 10 million joules (actually 10,450,000 joules). It's therefore more convenient to talk in kilojoules (1 kilojoule = 1,000 joules). That means that we take in – and lose – about 10,000 kilojoules per day in round figures.

Joules are more fundamental because they are linked to other fundamental units. Expending energy at 1 joule per second is called 1 watt. A little calculation shows that 10,000 kilojoules expended over twenty-four hours is a little over 100 watts, so we humans expend energy rather like a bright old-fashioned incandescent light bulb.

Other abbreviations that I will use for units are kg for kilograms (1 kg = 1,000 grams).

2

Human energy balance measurements: Firm foundations

A few years ago, we swapped our diesel-powered car for a fully electric model. We have solar photovoltaic panels on the roof of our house. When the sun shines, I get a schoolboyish delight in connecting the car to our smart charging point and watching it charge with power that's coming straight from the sun. When we go out for a drive, it's fun knowing that we are solar-powered.

Let's think through what's going on here. Nuclear reactions in the sun are liberating energy. This comes to earth as light energy. My roof panels convert a fraction of that (around 20 per cent) to electrical energy. That goes into the car battery. When we drive the car, say to our local garden centre, the electrical energy is converted to movement – which means acceleration of the car, giving it kinetic energy, overcoming air resistance and the resistance of the tyres on the road. When I slow the car down, some of that kinetic energy is cleverly converted back into electrical energy, but all the rest, along with the work done against air and road resistance, is lost as heat.

We see the conversion of energy between different forms.

And the human body also takes in energy – as we saw in the previous chapter, chemical energy in food and drink – and converts it to other forms of energy, mostly heat and perhaps some external work. If more energy is taken in than is used, there will be an increase in the body's energy stores. That bit can't be controversial, I hope. The real issue is, perhaps, whether we can really measure energy in, energy out, and – what might seem the most problematic part – quantify other routes for the energy to get lost, such as the residues that pass through us and are expelled in urine and faeces. And then, whether we can relate any differences to changes in body energy stores and, ultimately, weight.

What would we expect to see, on the basis of the energy balance model, if we were to study human energy intake and expenditure? I think it's reasonable to say that if we study someone who has a generally steady weight, we should expect his or her energy intake to match energy expenditure, although not necessarily on a day-to-day basis but certainly when averaged over periods of perhaps a week or two or three. And if intake and expenditure don't match, we would expect a change in body weight that relates to the difference between them – again, on a reasonably long-term basis.

This is all experimentally testable. And, indeed, it has been tested, extensively, for more than a century. But while the early experiments seemed to fully support the energy balance model, later research began to throw doubts upon it. And I believe that those doubts have led, in part, to today's questioning of the model.

How do we measure energy expended?

As we have seen, energy expenditure is reflected in the heat lost by the body (plus any external work done, such as moving or lifting objects). This is the principle that was used to measure the energy expenditure of small animals, such as guinea pigs, by Lavoisier and other scientists in the late eighteenth century: direct measurement of the heat lost from the body. Measurement of heat, a form of energy, is called 'calorimetry'. When we measure heat loss from the body directly it is called 'direct calorimetry'.

As we also saw, however, Lavoisier was able to measure the amount of oxygen used by a human body (that of his assistant Séguin) as a reflection of his oxidation of nutrients. In the following century, as precise values could be attached to the use of different fuels, it became possible to use oxygen consumption indirectly to measure energy expenditure. (A small improvement is made if production of carbon dioxide is also measured. Or carbon dioxide production alone can be used.) This method of assessing heat production, or energy expenditure, by measuring the use of oxygen or production of carbon dioxide is known as 'indirect calorimetry'. Direct calorimetry for humans is fraught with technical difficulties, and has now largely been replaced by indirect calorimetry.[1] Around the time of the Second World War, small devices were developed that could be worn in a backpack, to sample expired breath and collect samples for later laboratory analysis. This enabled a growing science of energy expenditure measurements during various recreational and occupational activities. Energy expenditure measurements began to become part of the assessment of training for elite athletes, and also hospital assessment of patients, especially in testing for thyroid disease. Modern indirect calorimetry instruments usually use either a soft mask that is strapped on the subject's face to collect breath via a flexible hose, or a clear plastic hood that goes over the head of a subject, lying in bed at rest, and through which air is drawn and collected for analysis.

Both techniques, direct and indirect calorimetry, have been

fundamental to the study of human energy balance. They are excellent for studying people in laboratory conditions, or under close supervision, but they can't tell us anything about how much energy you or I expend during our normal daily lives. For completeness here, we will jump ahead to a further development in measuring human energy expenditure, the so-called 'doubly labelled water method'. This was introduced for human studies in 1982 by Dale Schoeller and E. van Santen at the University of Chicago.[2] Its big advantage is that the subject of the measurement does not need to be confined to a small chamber. For the subjects, it is very simple. They are given a glass of special water to drink, and then they collect small samples of urine or saliva over the next two to three weeks. The trick is that the water, H_2O, is 'labelled' with special atoms (isotopes) of hydrogen and oxygen (hence, 'doubly labelled water'). By tracking how fast these isotopes disappear from the body, the experimenter can calculate the rate at which the person is breathing out carbon dioxide. As we have seen, this reflects the rate of energy expenditure. This technique has fundamentally changed our ideas of energy balance under different conditions, as we will see in later chapters.

Setting the scene: early human energy balance studies

Much of European biological science in the nineteenth century was concerned with improving the growth of farm animals. Schools of agriculture were established, and the fundamentals of animal nutrition were discovered: that carbohydrates, fats and proteins supply energy, and that protein is necessary, in particular, for growth.[3] At the same time, there was continuing interest in understanding the 'origins of animal heat' – what happens inside the body that led to Lavoisier's conclusions about metabolism. The French Académie des Sciences offered a prize for the 'Determination of the source of animal heat', leading to further measurements on small animals such as rabbits.[4] Then the German chemist Carl von Voit in Munich and his students, Max Rubner and Max von Pettenkofer, developed larger instruments. Pettenkofer is generally credited with building the first indirect calorimeter for humans – then called a respiration calorimeter – for studying human energy expenditure, in the 1860s. Funding was provided by the enlightened King Maximilian II of Bavaria.[5] (The scientists of this time were extremely versatile. Pettenkofer's Wikipedia entry describes his work on hygiene and public health with hardly a mention of his work in nutrition, and nothing on his work on calorimetry. He had a special interest in cholera.[6]) Pettenkofer's respiration calorimeter consisted of a small room in which a person could stay for some hours, and which was ventilated by air that then passed into an instrument that measured how much carbon dioxide had been produced. He studied men at rest, after feeding and during exercise. His experiments all confirmed the idea that the human body uses three fuels – carbohydrates, fats and proteins – to liberate energy by combining them with oxygen, the process of oxidation. His colleague Rubner, meanwhile, in parallel studies, showed that any one of these three fuels could supply the energy for metabolism, the amount each supplied being equivalent to the heat released when it was burned in the laboratory – this became known as the 'isodynamic law': 'that the food-stuffs may under given conditions replace each other in accordance with their heat-producing value'. He determined values of 4.1 kcal per gram of carbohydrate, 9.3 kcal per gram of fat, and 4.1 kcal per gram of protein, values very close to those commonly used today.[7] In 1885, after moving to Marburg, Rubner also built a calorimeter inside which a dog could live for extended periods. Over forty-five days, he determined that the dog's total heat production was 17,350 kcal, and energy expenditure calculated from the respiratory metabolism (oxygen consumption and carbon dioxide production) was 17,410 kcal – amazingly close agreement, given that they were completely independent methods of measurement.[8]

Confirmation of the validity of the energy balance model applied to humans, though, required a larger calorimeter. Wilbur Atwater, an American agricultural chemist, who had been an undergraduate during the American Civil War, spent two periods in Germany, on the second occasion having obtained a grant to determine whether humans could digest fish equally well as meat. He worked with von Voit in Munich, and also toured around Europe looking at how agricultural research had developed. Back in the USA, he urged the US government to create its own agricultural research stations. In 1887, he was appointed director of the experimental station that was established at Storrs Agricultural College, Connecticut, and here he began the work for which he is nowadays best known on human energy balance.[9]

Atwater worked with Edward Rosa, a physicist and engineer, at the Wesleyan University at Middletown, Connecticut to build a calorimeter in which human volunteers could be studied.[10] It consisted of a chamber measuring 2.1 × 1.2 metres floor space, 1.9 metres high, described by the experimenters as:

> an air-tight copper box, surrounded by zinc and wooden walls with air spaces between ... large enough for a man to remain in it in comfort for a number of days. A ventilating current of air is pumped through the chamber at such a rate that the subject can always be supplied with a sufficiency of pure air. The chamber contains a folding bed, chair, table, etc., and is provided with means for the introduction of food and drink and the removal of excreta.[11]

Water ran in pipes through the walls. As the human volunteer inside liberated heat, so this raised the temperature of the water leaving the calorimeter, and the difference in temperature could be measured to assess heat production. In addition, as this was also a respiration calorimeter, carbon dioxide production (and, later, oxygen consumption) were measured from changes in the air as it passed through the chamber.

This simple description, however, belies the almost unbelievable technical difficulty of the measurements: so many different variables needed to be accounted for – just, for example, the heat lost by evaporation of water in expired breath. Indeed, there is a note in their report about their use of a bomb calorimeter (described below), not just for analysing the foods provided but also for analysing 'liquid and solid excreta', as the experimenters delicately described them. It is now generally accepted that these investigators, with their attention to detail, obtained results to a degree of accuracy that has not been matched since.

The human calorimeter was constructed over several years, starting in 1892. Rosa moved away from the project in around 1899,[12] and Atwater then worked with nutritionist Francis Benedict, later well known in the metabolic community for his work on human starvation[13] (we shall discuss this work again in later chapters). Descriptions of the calorimeter, and the results of the experiments, were published as a series of reports in the Year Book of the US Department of Agriculture, and in the journal *Physical Review*. The longest of these reports, at nearly 400 pages, by Atwater and Benedict, dated 1903,[14] describes a series of twenty-one experiments conducted between 1900 and 1902 – an experiment was typically one subject studied for four whole days in the chamber. Much of the report concerns experimental methods. The calibration of the instrumentation was regularly checked using two different approaches. An electric heater in the chamber was used to generate a known amount of heat, to check that this was accurately captured. In addition, known amounts of alcohol were burned, to check that the expected use of oxygen and the production of carbon dioxide were found. All these checks, and their results, are tabulated in detail in the report, as are chemical analyses, including 'heat of combustion' measured in the bomb calorimeter, of all the foodstuffs provided for the volunteers, and all the volunteers' excreta.

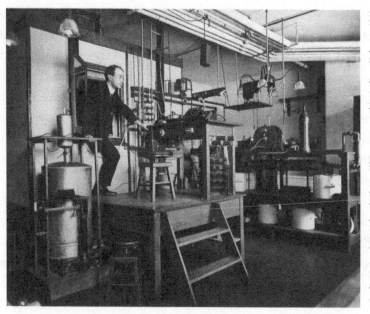

Credit: National Agricultural Library, US Department of Agriculture, Unknown 1910

A volunteer emerging from the hatch of the Atwater calorimeter (astonishingly, to present-day eyes, dressed in suit and tie).

The bomb calorimeter was a key tool used by these investigators. Atwater had seen this in use in Rubner's laboratory. This is the instrument used to measure the heat released when a substance is burned. It consists of a strong steel inner container in which the substance to be analysed is held in an atmosphere of oxygen under high pressure, and with an electrical filament to start combustion. Heat is measured by surrounding this 'bomb' with water held in a larger, insulated container, and measuring the change in temperature of the water. It is the method used to measure the energy content of foods, then and even nowadays. Atwater used it both for analysing the energy content of all foods supplied to the experimental subjects within the chamber, and for assessing energy lost in urine and faeces. (Since liquid urine would not 'burn', it was absorbed into a block of cellulose, dried and combusted: the heat of combustion of the same amount of cellulose had been measured separately.)[15]

That 1903 report describes the 'primary object' of the experiments as 'the study of metabolism of matter and energy in the living organism', and among questions addressed is 'the proof that the law of the conservation of energy obtains in the body'. That's just what we want to establish. Their accuracy of measurement got better as they became more familiar with adjustments to the instrument.[16] The temperature of water entering the heat-exchange system was continually adjusted by an external assistant, warmer water being supplied for a subject at rest than when the volunteer was exercising, in order to keep the temperature within the chamber constant. A rather striking statement from the 1904 report[17] shows just how sensitive the measurements of heat released could be. They report that 'During the period of deep sleep the subject ordinarily gives off heat from the body at the rate of 60 to 75 calories per hour, or enough to raise the temperature of 1.3 to 1.7 pounds [0.6 to 0.8 kg] of water from freezing to boiling ... ' (For calories here, read kcal.) And because of that, 'any slight temporary rise in the temperature of the chamber like that which would result from an increase in heat production because of movement of the subject, such as rising from his chair, stretching out the arms, or moving in bed, can be at once detected by the observer ... ' In fact, the heat produced by a human body at rest over twenty-four hours is enough to raise the temperature of around 25 kg of water from freezing to boiling point – this may seem rather remarkable, but it makes the measurement of instantaneous heat production feasible.

Atwater and Benedict later summarised the results of '45 metabolism experiments covering 143 experimental days'. The experimental days included periods of exercise as well as rest, and periods of 'special diet' as well as 'normal diet'. The data are astonishing. The daily figures for energy input (food and drink) and heat loss (energy expenditure), averaged over these forty-five experiments, were respectively 3,481 kcal and (almost unbelievably) 3,481 kcal.[18] Remember that these two figures were based upon entirely separate measurements.

By the time of their final report, dated 1905, Atwater and Benedict had been able to calculate the changes in body stores of carbohydrate, fat and protein from their careful analyses of what was taken in and what came out, including measurements of oxygen consumption, carbon dioxide production and the balance of nitrogen in and out. They show an example of an experiment in which they calculated the balance of each nutrient – carbohydrate, fat and protein – in a subject followed for five days in the calorimeter, and from this predicted the change in body weight to be a fall of 118 grams. In fact, the drop in body weight measured directly was 111 grams.[19] They seem slightly disappointed with this discrepancy, and state that: 'Subsequent experience with the platform balance has shown that with a perfected technique the agreement between the computed gain or loss of body material and that actually found is very close.' They then compared their calculation of the heat that should have been liberated from the oxidation of the food taken in (allowing for energy lost in urine and faeces) and the change in body stores, with the heat measured directly as heat output. The figures are respectively 2,090 kcal and 2,110 kcal, a discrepancy of 1.6 per cent, which, considering all the measurements involved, is pretty impressive.[20]

Energy values of nutrients and foods

As part of his work on human energy balance, Atwater needed to determine the energy values (the heat released when burned) of the foods that were fed to the volunteers in the calorimeters. He realised that there is a difference between the energy released when the whole foodstuff is burned, and the energy that the body could obtain from it, as some would pass straight through. This is why he and his colleagues also analysed energy in faeces and urine (although there was very little in urine). The difference gave what is generally now called 'metabolisable energy' – Atwater referred to this as 'digestibility'. It is important to say that for most foods, only a small proportion of their energy passes through in faeces, although for plant materials with what we would now call a 'high fibre content' (Atwater termed this 'refuse', along with bones, eggshells, and so on) that proportion is generally larger. In a tabulation of the digestibility, nutrient by nutrient, in a range of foods, he found carbohydrates in animal products (not that there is much) to be 98 per cent digestible, 90–98 per cent for carbohydrates in vegetable products, and 97 per cent in a mixed diet. For fats the values were, respectively, 95, 90 and (mixed diet) 95 per cent, and protein was 97 per cent digestible in animal products, but less in those of vegetable origin (80–90 per cent): Atwater suggested a figure of 92 per cent digestibility for the protein of a mixed diet.[21] We shall revisit this issue in a later chapter, as we now understand much more about what happens to the 'refuse' in our large intestine, and how this might be changed.

Atwater observed that the energy values of individual nutrients varied. They varied according to the food from which they were obtained, and also he noted that different carbohydrates (for example, starches and simple sugars) gave slightly different values. But, understanding the need for practical advice, he generalised over a range of foods and, taking digestibility into account, came up with the figures of 4.0 kcal per gram for carbohydrates, 8.9 kcal per gram for fats (now usually taken as 9 kcal per gram), and 4.0 kcal per gram for protein: values that are still widely used today, often known as the 'Atwater Factors'.[22]

The data collected on different foods by Atwater and his colleague Arthur Bryant were published in 1906. They listed data for 4,000 foods, many analysed by themselves, but also including other researchers' results.[23] Such was the importance of Atwater's work as a nutritional scientist, and also as a manager of agricultural research in the USA, that the British nutritionist Elsie Widdowson (whom we are about to get to know more closely) wrote: 'I think I can safely say that Atwater has contributed more to our knowledge about the assessment of the energy value of human foods than anyone who has ever lived, either before or since his time.'[24]

Later in the twentieth century, two British nutritionists began similar work. Robert McCance had been a Royal Navy pilot in the First World War, bravely flying from a wooden platform over the gun turret of a warship. Later, he studied medicine in London, and was offered a research position by R.D. Lawrence, one of the UK pioneers of the treatment of diabetes. Lawrence wanted better analyses of the carbohydrate content of vegetables – until then, Atwater's method of measuring carbohydrate 'by difference' had been used (carbohydrate was taken as the difference in weight between the whole food and the measured protein, fat and mineral contents). This work broadened in scope to include other foods and nutrients, and McCance was joined at King's College in London by nutritionist Elsie Widdowson.[25] In 1940 they published the first version of their food tables as *The*

Composition of Foods. This database has been updated many times over the intervening years and is currently available in book form and as a searchable database, now called *McCance and Widdowson's The Composition of Foods.*[26] It underpins almost all dietary research in the UK and Europe. Widdowson worked for much of her career in Cambridge, having moved there when McCance was made Professor of Experimental Medicine. She is regarded by British nutritionists today as a key figure in understanding the nutritional requirements for growth. But it is her work on energy balance in adults that is relevant to this story.[27]

Getting a handle on human energy requirements

It seems clear, then, that when volunteers are confined to a calorimeter, fed meals of precisely known composition, and are doing known amounts of exercise, the principle of energy balance can be shown to apply to humans as closely as it does to smaller animals. But this proved little about how we behave outside the confines of a laboratory. Trying to understand this conundrum occupied researchers for much of the second half of the last century.

The work of McCance and Widdowson on food composition started because of the need to better understand human energy requirements in wartime. During the Second World War, food for civilians in many countries, including the UK, was strictly rationed. The government needed to know whether these rations were sufficient. The armed forces needed to know how much energy was needed by those in active service. After the war, people who had been starved or underfed during the war needed refeeding. Many nutritional scientists contributed to understanding these topics.

Ancel Keys, in Minnesota, USA, conducted a long-term study of underfeeding and then refeeding in a group of Conscientious Objectors. This work, generally known as the Minnesota Experiment, has been written about extensively, and we shall look at data from it in later chapters.[28] McCance and Widdowson were involved in similar work. They looked at the effects of wartime rationing, conducting many studies, mainly on themselves, to see if they could remain healthy on the restricted diets offered to the civilian population. Indeed, together with the physiologist Andrew Huxley,* they hiked together for ten days in the snowy English Lake District, covering up to 36 miles per day, eating mainly bread, cabbage and potatoes.[29]

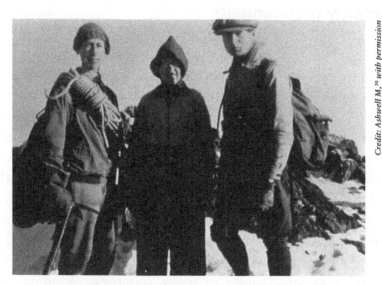

Credit: Ashwell M,[30] with permission

Robert McCance (left), Elsie Widdowson and the physiologist Andrew Huxley, in the English Lake District during their experiments on rationing, 1940.

---

* Later awarded the 1963 Nobel Prize in physiology or medicine for his work on nerve impulses.

They did all this while continuing to collaborate on their food tables, which were progressively updated. In the 1950s, though, they turned their attention directly to human energy balance: studies that, as we shall see in the next chapter, had a profound influence on the unease with which some now regard the principle of 'calories in–calories out'. These formed part of a series of studies by British nutritionists and physiologists, covering the period from the early 1950s to 1970, directly addressing questions of energy balance. Some of these have formed part of the folklore of the field, and we will look at them here and in the next chapter as they give us clear pointers as to why the concept of energy balance can be so problematic.

Reg Passmore – a name we will meet several times in this context – was a medically qualified physiologist and nutritionist, known to many students of dietetics through his textbook *Human Nutrition and Dietetics*. During the Second World War, he worked in the Indian Medical Service and gained experience of dealing with malnutrition as well as infectious diseases and wartime wounds. Later, he conducted research at the University of Edinburgh, and collaborated closely with John Durnin of the Institute of Physiology at the University of Glasgow.[31] They are joint authors of a fascinating little book, *Energy, Work and Leisure* (1967), in which they collated the many measurements they had made of energy expenditure in various industrial and sporting activities, mostly using a backpack instrument to collect expired air for later analysis in the laboratory. Passmore published in 1952 the results of a detailed energy balance study in a small group of students.[32] These students were clearly very cooperative and, as the authors describe:

> The problem of recording, from minute to minute and from day to day for 13 days, the multifarious activities of five

active young men seemed, on first consideration, to demand the assistance of five observers. Under other conditions, with less intelligent or less enthusiastically co-operative subjects this is probably so. In the present investigation, however, each subject acted as his own observer, timing and recording his activities in great detail on a specially designed activity chart.

These young volunteers were studied over one week during rest and physical activity. They each tabulated all their food and drink in detail. Their energy expenditure during activities was measured with the device worn in a backpack: at rest, it was measured with a stand-alone apparatus. The paper makes clear the difficulties of doing such experiments. We are told that on one afternoon 'conditions [outside] were so bad that climbing up and down stairs in the laboratory was substituted for walking'. Further, 'three of the subjects developed blisters and minor orthopaedic trouble which on occasions restricted activity', and to complicate matters more:

> John, one of the fittest, developed mumps in the middle of the experiment and was only available for heavy work on 3 days, during which he walked 50 miles. Evan, whose feet prevented his exercising on one day, walked 52 miles. Iain, George and Alistair walked 66, 71 and 76 miles respectively, spread out over the 5-day period.

The long-suffering volunteers were clearly highly motivated to make this study a success. Despite all the problems, the authors were able to show a close agreement between energy intake and expenditure, with small differences reflected in changes in body weight, as we would expect from the principle of energy balance.

Another example comes from a study published in 1962 by Nan Taggart, a researcher in Aberdeen with an interest in pregnancy and nutrition.[33] She describes detailed observations on 'a 31-year-old woman'; Durnin and Passmore, in their book *Energy, Work and Leisure*, suggest that this was, indeed, the author herself. The subject of the observations was meticulous in recording everything relevant, including, for example, weighing herself, dressed, in the laboratory on arrival in the morning – having taken the precaution of weighing her clothes at home before dressing. She ate her breakfast after weighing. She weighed all her food and drink before consuming it, to an accuracy of 2 grams. She kept records over two periods: the first period of eighty days finished in late December (26th) and she delayed eating her Christmas dinner until after that, in order to avoid anything unusual. During this first period she ate normally and exercised as she normally would, but during the second period of thirty-five days she tried to keep food intake and activity constant from day to day. Her meticulous records show energy intake varying considerably from day to day, but with a very consistent pattern: lower during the working week, and higher at weekends, peaking each Sunday. Her weight fluctuated by almost 1 kg from day to day in the first period but was much steadier (daily variations of less than 0.5 kg) in the second period. Her body weight in the first period was linked to her energy intake in a broad sense, peaking at weekends, although from beginning to end of the eighty days it had not changed. Taggart measured water balance by collecting and measuring all fluid intake and urine excretion, and she showed that the fluctuations in weight were, in fact, more closely related to fluid than to energy balance. This is a crucial observation, one that has big implications for all dieters.

The nature of our fuel stores confounds energy balance studies

The experiments detailed above all looked at how we expend energy, but how is it stored? This is complex, with different stores used over different time periods, and, as Nan Taggart surmised, it confounds short-term measures of energy balance and weight. We store carbohydrate as the starch-like substance called 'glycogen', in our muscle and liver cells, but this store is small in extent. Glycogen in the liver is sufficient to keep the brain supplied with glucose – usually its major fuel – for about twenty-four hours. Muscle glycogen is there mainly to fuel muscle contraction, although it is indeed consumed when we are not eating – there are not good data for this in humans, but it has been estimated that muscle glycogen would be depleted within a week or so of starvation.[34] Our glycogen stores total something under 1 kg when we are well fed. But much more importantly, from the point of view of body-weight changes, is that glycogen, being a starchy substance, is always associated with water. One kg of glycogen will be stored with around 3 kg of water; and when glycogen is used, this water is lost into the bloodstream and ultimately into the urine.

By far our major energy store, used for longer-term needs, is in the form of fat. In people of normal weight, this is almost entirely stored in the specialised tissue called 'adipose tissue' under the skin. (As we lay down more fat, it might be stored within the abdomen, in and around our organs, and this is associated with ill health.) Fat can be stored with very little added water. What is more, fat, when oxidised, liberates more than twice the energy (gram for gram) of carbohydrates such as glycogen, as Rubner and then Atwater had shown. We may carry around many kilograms of fat. An average figure among 1,500 people randomly recruited from the Oxfordshire population was 25 kg.*[35] (Out of interest, the lowest fat mass among this group was 6 kg, the greatest 68 kg – a more than ten-fold range. This just shows how widely it may vary from person to person.) Twenty-five kg of fat would be sufficient to keep us alive for a matter of months if we ate nothing else.

Here is the difficulty, though, that we will consider again when we think about attempts to lose weight. When we re-strict our energy intake, the first thing to change appreciably is the glycogen store, with its water: so, pronounced shifts of a small number of kilograms can occur quickly, which do not for the most part reflect energy stores – they are mostly water. This is sometimes called 'water weight'. John Garrow illus-trates this clearly with the results of an experiment in which a volunteer (whose name is not disclosed, but was almost certainly himself) was fed meals of disguised energy content over a ten-day period. The subject was weighed twice each day and his energy balance was monitored closely. When the energy imbalance for each half-day was plotted against the change in weight (measured under very consistent conditions), a remarkably strong relationship appeared. Each 100 kcal of energy imbalance (whether a surplus or deficit of energy) was reflected in a change in weight (up or down) of 100 grams. As Garrow points out, this is exactly what would be expected if these short-term energy imbalances are reflected in changes in the store of glycogen (4 kcal per gram) with its associated water (around 3 grams to each gram of glycogen).[36] Only in the longer term are our fat stores relevant to studies of energy balance – and they change by much less because they represent such a dense form of energy.

Similarly, a small surplus of energy intake over expenditure

---

* The Oxford BioBank is a database of people in the local population main-tained by my colleague Prof Fredrik Karpe, who kindly arranged for me to have data on 1,500 randomly selected people. We will use these data again in later chapters.

will result in a rapid rebuilding of the glycogen stores – with associated water. This is one of the difficulties faced by the dieter: the least transgression of the daily energy targets will result in rapid weight gain, and potentially despair, although what the scales are measuring is mostly water. Reg Passmore, reviewing this field in 1967, considered this. He reckoned that measurement of body fat (which, because of these shifts in fluid balance, will give a more accurate picture of energy stores than body weight) was at best correct to within 1 kg, meaning that 'measurements of body fat are therefore quite useless in energy balance studies in humans, unless the calorie imbalance is large, probably of the order of 20,000 kcal. This means in practice that the study must be continued over at least 4 weeks ...'[37] (We will look in Chapter 7 at methods for measuring body fat in humans.) Here, then, we see yet another difficulty in appreciating the link between energy balance and body weight. We shall shortly learn that this is but one of many factors persuading so many people that calories in–calories out is not a useful way to think of weight regulation.

We have looked at the early studies that confirm the fundamentals of human energy balance. I have cherry-picked some later studies in which these principles were tested in people outside the close confines of a laboratory – studies that seem to confirm that human energy balance behaves just as we might expect from the laws of physics. A characteristic of these studies is that the experimental volunteers were themselves closely involved in the studies: Passmore's long-suffering and sore-footed young men, or Nan Taggart herself. In the next chapter, though, we will see how this has not always been the case: and we shall begin to see where the difficulties lie in believing in the basic idea of calories in–calories out and its relationship to our body-weight trajectory.

3

Human energy balance measurements: Perhaps it's not so simple

By the early part of the last century, then, scientists had good reason to believe that human energy balance behaved as we would expect from the laws of physics – and could be shown experimentally to do so, at least when people were studied under very controlled conditions. But, as studies of energy balance were expanded beyond these rather artificial constraints, difficulties began to arise: difficulties that I believe are at the heart of present dissatisfaction with the energy balance model. Looking at why these difficulties arose will lead us into a deep consideration of the experimental problems of assessing energy balance in anyone but a volunteer under very close scrutiny.

Audits of human energy balance

In the early 1950s, the staff of a training establishment for young soldiers in the UK consulted the physiologist Otto

Edholm. The general who had inspected the cadets felt that they were not gaining weight as they should because they were not getting enough 'good red meat' to cover their very active lifestyle. He asked Edholm to investigate. Edholm went to see Robert McCance and Elsie Widdowson, and they took up the challenge together.[1]

Edholm had an unusual background. He was born in London to Swedish parents, trained in medicine but specialised in physiological research. During the Second World War he worked with the UK's Medical Research Council Shock Committee on the problems of haemorrhage – as might occur in wounded soldiers – and blood-pressure control. (This was 'shock' as in traumatic shock – the same problem I was involved in, from a metabolic point of view, later in Manchester.) After the war, he was appointed Professor of Physiology at the Royal Veterinary College in London, where he and his associates worked on the venous valves in the giraffe, the okapi, the camel and the ostrich; then, in 1947 Edholm took the chair of physiology in the University of Western Ontario, and it was during his stay in Canada that he became interested in the effects on the body of extreme conditions. By this time, it was clear that the armed services would have to adapt to extremes of temperature and climatic conditions, and the Medical Research Council decided to set up a division of human physiology at the National Institute for Medical Research in London with a primary remit to study adaptation to cold. Edholm returned to the UK in 1949 to head this division and supervise the building of the unique climatic chambers at the Institute.[2] His later work included studies of the physiology of people swimming the English Channel, approximately 34 km of open water, and of polar explorers. This gave him expertise in measuring energy expenditure during various types of extreme activity, which would complement the expertise of Widdowson and McCance in assessing energy intake.

These three scientists, then, decided to approach the problem of whether the cadets were being adequately fed by conducting an audit of energy intake and expenditure, just as Passmore did for his small group of students. The first results from this study were published in 1954.[3]

The researchers set out to document the food and drink, and hence energy intake, and the energy expenditure of seventy-seven cadets 'aged 18½ to 20 years at one of the training establishments for the armed forces'. (The establishment is not named in their papers, but Widdowson lets slip in a personal account that it was the Royal Military Academy, Sandhurst, the training centre for new officers.[4]) One group of observers recorded what the men ate. Another observed what they did, and hence, using previously measured values for energy expenditure in various activities, calculated their energy expenditure. Although the inspecting general had imagined that these young men were vigorously active during their training, in fact Widdowson and her colleagues noted, a little disparagingly, that 'the cadets spent 9¼ h a day sitting, some of it at lectures, and 8½ h in bed. Dressing and cleaning uniform occupied more of their time and energy than sport or military training.' The average daily energy intake of the cadets was 3,710 kcal, and their energy expenditure 3,420 kcal. The authors commented, again a little acerbically, that these figures were considerably lower than reported energy intakes 'for American university football players (5,600 kcal/day) or for Olympic athletes (7,300 kcal/day)'.

This study was conducted over one week in 1952, and no attempt was made to look at differences between the individual cadets, nor to assess the effects of the apparent energy imbalance. (The authors acknowledged that this might have reflected under-estimation of energy expenditure.) In 1953 the same group of researchers decided to try to improve the measurements, especially those of energy expenditure, by including more direct measurements of oxygen consumption; and they hoped to be able to look in more detail at differences between individuals. The results of these studies, now conducted over two weeks, were reported by Edholm and the others in 1955.[5] Twelve of the young men were studied in detail.

Now, over a fortnight and with these improved methods, there was good agreement between the average values for daily energy intake (3,430 kcal) and energy expenditure (3,420 kcal). But those mean figures hid big variations, both from day to day within each individual, and between individuals. The authors presented a graph, a scattergram, showing the daily energy expenditure plotted against energy intake for each of the twelve cadets – so there were 168 points (12 × 14), forming what looks like a random cloud. There was clearly no relationship between one day's intake and that day's energy expenditure, as measured in this study. Daily energy intake ranged from just over 2,000 kcal to just under 5,000 kcal, whereas daily expenditure ranged from 2,300 to 5,600 kcal: big ranges. There was, as the authors put it, 'no correlation between the mean expenditure on any one day and the intake on that day', although, interestingly, when they plotted each against time, there appeared to be a lag of two days before energy intake matched expenditure – as though there were some mechanism by which expenditure was remembered and then, later, intake changed to match.

This study therefore gave no real support to the idea of energy balance, or certainly that it might be predicted in any way, or that it followed any rules that might be useful to the nutritionist – at least in the relatively short term.

John Durnin in Glasgow pursued these studies, looking for some pattern.[6] He collated data from studies on sixty-nine individuals in six groups, including, in the language of the time, groups of 'middle-aged housewives', of 'male office clerks', of 'coal-face miners', two separate groups of younger people – and the group of twelve military cadets reported by Edholm in 1955. Each of the individuals had been studied for (at least) one week so that there were seven consecutive daily determinations of energy intake and energy expenditure on each subject. As we have seen for the cadets, food intake was measured by 'the individual inventory method', that is by listing what was eaten, and the expenditure of energy, by asking the subjects to complete diaries of activity, and attributing energy costs to the various activities. Durnin postulated that, if the human body is striving to maintain a balance of energy intake and expenditure, he should find some relationship between these two variables when comparing one day with another for the same individual. In fact, out of the sixty-nine people studied, a statistically significant correlation between the two variables was found in only ten; and, among those, four showed a negative correlation – that is, they tended to show less energy intake on days when expenditure was high. Probably nowadays we would look at these data and say that it could all have been down to chance. Durnin, try as he might, was unable to provide convincing evidence that the volunteers' energy intake and expenditure were matched in any consistent way.

Otto Edholm persisted, however. By the late 1960s he felt that methodology had improved to the extent that it would be worth repeating the study on army cadets. In particular, one of his colleagues, Heinz Wolff, had designed a new instrument for collecting expired air to measure oxygen consumption, which sampled breath at intervals and saved the samples for later analysis. This machine was called the Integrating Motor Pneumotachograph (IMP): its inventor introduced the term 'bioengineering' and went on to become not just an important figure in that field, but also a popular television presenter of science topics. The sixty-four cadets now studied by Edholm carried this IMP on their backs during many of their activities.

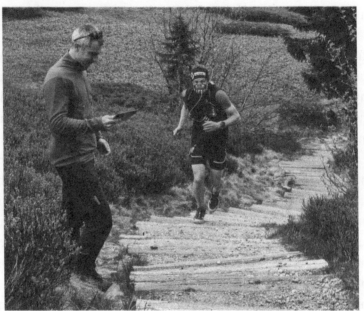

Credit: Cortex Biophysik, courtesy of Mrs Viviane Nagel

Measuring energy expenditure during activity with a backpack apparatus. Shown here is the Cortex Metamax instrument, which conducts real-time analyses of oxygen and carbon dioxide in breath. Previous generations of these instruments, such as the IMP described above, collected small samples of breath for later analysis.

To use Edholm's own description, when he published the results in 1970, 'since they ate in a common dining hall, and had almost identical activities, they were suitable subjects in whom to study calorie balance'. As well as measurement of energy expenditure using the IMP, detailed observations and diaries were also kept of their activities. They were fed 'already weighed meals' and 'an observer measured the bread, butter and tea consumed and weighed the plate waste, separating it into its components'. The volunteers were also weighed ('nude, after urinating') daily. The detailed work that went into the measurements is clear.

When Edholm analysed the results, however, they were again confusing. On a day-to-day basis, there was no relationship between energy intake and energy expenditure. The volunteers had been studied at six different centres in England and Wales. At half the centres, he found some relationship between the food energy taken in over the three-week period of the study and the energy expended, but at the other three there was no relationship at all. When he looked at 'calorie balance' over the experimental period (that is, the difference between energy taken in and energy expended) it was mostly positive: more energy taken in than expended. These army cadets were being well fed. And, as we would expect, most gained some weight. But there was little relationship between the two measurements, and he noted that 'nine subjects gained a good deal more [weight] than their calorie balance would seem to justify'.[7]

By this time there was growing international interest in nutritional issues for people in low-income countries, many of whom were still undernourished. There was a need to understand human energy requirements in order to provide appropriate nutritional support. Four very eminent British nutritionists and physiologists, including Edholm and Durnin, wrote on this topic for the journal *Nature* in 1973. The other authors were Derek Miller of Queen Elizabeth College, University of London and John Waterlow of the London School of Hygiene and Tropical Medicine. Each of these figures carried considerable weight in the field of human physiology, nutrition and dietetics. They stated that:

We believe that the energy requirements of man and his balance of intake and expenditure are not known.

Paradoxically, we conclude this from results of the increasingly sophisticated studies of food intake and energy expenditure which show that in any group of twenty or more subjects, with similar attributes and activities, food intake can vary as much as two-fold. In those surveys where both intake and expenditure are measured, there is often good agreement between the two estimates for the average of the group, but usually very large discrepancies between individual intake and individual expenditure.[8]

By the early 1970s, the idea that energy intakes or expenditures were in any sense predictable, or even that they bore any relationship to each other, was seriously in doubt. I would say that we now know that these well-intentioned scientists were wrong. But acceptance of that would take several more decades – and, indeed, as we have seen, acceptance even now has not been by any means universal.

In the light of the early calorimetry studies, seeming to confirm the energy balance model, how should we now interpret the studies of the second half of the twentieth century by Passmore, Widdowson, Edholm, Durnin and their colleagues? John Garrow analysed the studies on the military cadets at length in his book *Energy Balance and Obesity in Man* (first published in 1974). He made some interesting observations. He pointed out that 'Energy balance is difficult to study [in humans] because there is no prompt response to an acute imbalance' – because we have a large energy reserve. In that way, energy balance is quite unlike other well-understood physiological responses such as thirst in response to lack of fluid, or temperature regulation. Indeed, Garrow says, 'It is difficult to think of any other physiological quantity which is so loosely regulated.' Garrow was unwilling to admit to the possibility of major measurement errors, quite reasonably given that he would have known the investigators personally and appreciated the care that they had taken with the measurements. Now, with the benefit of several decades of further research into the difficulties of knowing just what anyone is eating or how much energy they are expending, I think that is a generous interpretation.

What is noticeable is that these investigators had far less control over what the army cadets ate and what they did, than did the researchers described in Chapter 2. They believed that they could record the cadets' food intake accurately, for example. But there are some clues in the text of the papers as to why this might not have been as straightforward as the investigators hoped. Widdowson describes how the cadets ate breakfast together in the dining room – but then during the morning the cadets could go to the canteen, which served 'cakes, buns, sausages, milk and various soft drinks'. Lunch was served in the dining room, but attendance was not compulsory, and at the same time the canteens (plural) were open where the cadets could choose food and drinks freely. Afternoon tea at 4pm was attended by about half the cadets, but once more the canteens were open as an alternative. There was a formal evening dinner, but on three days each week the canteens were open in the evening, and the cadets could also leave the campus and go outside. The paper admits that food and drink taken outside could not be so accurately assessed. We are about to learn just how little faith we should place on records of food consumption, particularly when, as I suspect may have been the case here, the recruits had no personal interest in the study – unlike the five students studied by Passmore and colleagues, and reported in 1952, or the single woman studied by Taggart, in whom agreement with the energy balance model seemed much more straightforward. We should also note Edholm's remark in the 1955 paper that 'There is a suggestion that for some reason the metabolic observations slightly reduced the intake of food. Both groups ate a little less during the weeks when the expenditures were being measured.' When, later, we look at research into the energy balance of people in the wider community, we shall see that the difficulties of knowing what any one person is doing are even greater.

Measuring energy intake – it's not as simple as it sounds

In the last chapter we looked briefly at methods for measuring energy expenditure. It's worth considering at this point how scientists measure energy intake, as this will have a bearing on much of the discussion to follow.

Suppose you were a volunteer in my research programme, and I needed to know what you eat. How would I get that information? There are a number of well-established methods for doing this. If you are not actually to come and live in my laboratory, the assessment would of necessity rely on your reporting what you eat. The most common method for doing this is to use a 'diet diary', in which the participant records all food eaten, usually with an assessment of the portion size. Sometimes, this is done for a few days: better estimates are obtained with a seven-day diary that includes a weekend. An experimenter, usually trained in nutrition and dietetics, will then enter all the information into a computer program, which will analyse what has been eaten and drunk in terms of energy and nutrients. Alternatively, a trained interviewer may ask the volunteer to recall all foods eaten in a preceding period, usually twenty-four hours. A related method for recording food intake is known as the Food Frequency Questionnaire. Volunteers are given a list of foods and asked to note how often they typically eat each of them. This is simpler for the volunteer, but generally less accurate than the food diary.

Methods such as these are used in large national surveys. In the USA, the CDC's National Health and Nutrition Examination Survey (NHANES) is 'a program of studies designed to assess the health and nutritional status of adults and children in the United States ... [which] began in the early 1960s and has been conducted as a series of surveys focusing on different population groups or health topics'.[9] NHANES includes measures of food intake. These are based upon interviews in which the subject is asked to remember what he or she has eaten over a 24-hour period. From 2002, a second dietary recall interview was added a few days later, after the participants had been given a booklet and some measuring guides.[10]

In the UK, the National Diet and Nutrition Survey (NDNS) 'is a continuous cross-sectional survey, jointly funded by Public Health England and the UK Food Standards Agency ... It is designed to assess the diet, nutrient intake and nutritional status of the general population aged 1.5 years and over living in private households in the UK.' As with the NHANES data, we looked at some of their information on energy intake over recent years in Chapter 1. For the years 2008 to 2019 dietary assessment was based on a food diary completed over four consecutive days. From 2020 onwards, the methodology has changed to 'a web-based automated self-administered 24-hour dietary recall tool. Participants are asked to record everything they ate and drank the previous day.'[11]

Just consider now how this works for a participant. On pages 54–55 you'll see part of a typical diet diary – this is the seven-day diary used in the European Prospective Investigation into Cancer (EPIC).

A seven-day food diary

| DATE | 2 | 3 | 1 | 0 | 1 | 9 | 9 | 3 | DAY OF WEEK | Saturday |

BEFORE BREAKFAST

Food/drink	Description/preparation	Amount
Orange squash	Robinsons Whole Orange – sweetened	1 glass

BREAKFAST

Food/drink	Description/preparation	Amount
Beef patty with onion	Homebaked cold Salt added	5oz
Tea	Typhoo	1 cup
Milk	Semi-skimmed	1 dessertspoon
Sugar	White	1½ teaspoons

MID MORNING – between breakfast and lunch time

Food/drink	Description/preparation	Amount
Coffee	Maxwell House instant ½ water, ½ semi-skimmed milk	1 mug
Sugar	White	1½ teaspoons
Cake	Homemade date cake	1 slice, 4oz

LUNCH		
Food/drink	Description/preparation	Amount
Gammon steak	Microwaved	6oz
Chips	Deep fried in oil (Crisp & Dry)	7oz
Peas	Birds Eye (frozen)	4 tablespoons
Bread	Local bakery, white unsliced	½ slice, thick
Apple pie	Homemade	4½ oz
Sugar	White - sprinkled on	1 teaspoon
Custard	Bird's - made with semi-skimmed milk	Small fruit dish

TEA - beween lunch and evening meal		
Food/drink	Description/preparation	Amount
Tea	Typhoo tea bag	1 mug
Milk	Semi-skimmed	1 dessertspoon
Sugar	White	1½ teaspoons
Biscuit	Fox's chocolate digestive	1

Credit: Medical Research council (MRC) Epidemiology Unit at the University of Cambridge, with permission

The drawbacks are obvious, however. I have on several occasions filled in diet diaries myself for the sake of our own research, usually for projects being run by students in the laboratory. I think I am generally an honest person, and it is in my interest to ensure that experimental results generated from my laboratory are as trustworthy as they can be. But even I cannot be sure I declared every last biscuit, or snippet of cheese, or little glass of wine before going to bed: I might not have wanted my students to know that. Even more importantly, of course, knowing that I was going to have to record the biscuit in the diary may well have meant that I decided not to eat it. The very act of recording my intake almost certainly influenced what I ate. It is a nutritional 'uncertainty principle'.

Only in controlled experimental situations – such as volunteers living within a calorimeter, and being fed by the experimenters – can we be sure of measuring energy intake accurately. If an experimental volunteer spends time in a research unit, the experimenters can measure what food is given to the volunteer, and what is left uneaten. But the situation of an experimenter determining exactly what the volunteer eats is unusual. It doesn't even answer one of the most common questions in nutrition: what does someone eat during their normal daily life?

We have some information on how accurate self-reporting of food intake is. During the 1970s and 1980s, the Medical Research Council's Dunn Clinical Nutrition Centre in Cambridge was a centre of nutritional and physiological research into obesity in the UK. It was becoming apparent to the scientists there, from a number of studies, that data on food and energy intake were not always reliable. The late Gail Goldberg, a young nutritional scientist working with others in the unit, began to analyse studies of energy intake, looking at how reported energy intake agreed with actual. 'Actual' in early studies was based on calculations of the known energy requirements for people of a similar body build. Goldberg showed that reported energy intake was often less than that required for survival. She then set limits on what would be believable figures for energy intake, based on the resting energy expenditure of subjects (which, if not reported, can be fairly accurately estimated from weight, height, sex and age), with allowances for additional energy expenditure during the day: as she put it, 'the fundamental principles of energy physiology'.[12] She applied this reasoning to '37 published dietary studies of adults providing 68 subgroups when classified according to sex and dietary method' (dietary method referred to whether the information was gathered by 'diet records, diet recall [or] diet history' – so covering all bases). The results were clear:

> When categorized according to dietary assessment method, 64%, 88% and 25% of results fell below the acceptable cut-off value for studies by diet records, diet recall and diet history, respectively. These data indicate that dietary assessment methods have a strong bias towards underestimation of habitual energy intake.[13]

Her method for assessing 'acceptable' energy intake is often now referred to as the Goldberg cut-off.

The conclusion that we all tend to under-report what we normally eat has been confirmed in many studies, including some detailed studies by Judith Hallfrisch and colleagues at the US Department of Agriculture's Beltsville Human Nutrition Research Center in Maryland. These investigators asked several hundred people to record their normal food intake, and also studied them in detail to determine their actual energy requirements. They found that 80 per cent of their participants reported their intake at 700 kcal/day below their maintenance requirement.[14]

Worse news, though, for the purposes of our understanding of body-weight regulation, is the finding (by Barbara Livingstone and Alison Black at the University of Ulster at Coleraine, Northern Ireland, reviewing this area in depth) that 'Profound underreporting was found in obese subjects ... A negative association between the extent of underreporting and measures of weight status (body weight, percentage body fat or BMI) has also been found in [many] studies ...' This means that the larger someone is, the more they tend to under-report energy intake.[15] Livingstone, with a Japanese colleague Kentaro Murakami, applied the 'Goldberg cut-off' analysis to data collected in the US NHANES study, on which much American nutritional advice is based. They again found under-reporting more prevalent, the more overweight were the subjects.[16] We shall look at this issue, which bedevils research into energy balance, again many times.

Yes, you might think: *but there must be better ways of recording what someone is eating using modern technology.* With the advent of mobile phones, it seems obvious that the experimenter might ask the volunteer to photograph what he or she is eating. This has been called 'image-assisted' or 'image-based dietary assessment'. In 2020, Dang Ho and colleagues from Taipei conducted a meta-analysis (a combination of published results) covering 606 participants. The results were no better: they found no statistical difference between image-based dietary assessments and 'traditional' methods. When measured energy intake was compared directly with measured energy expenditure (which should reflect energy intake), there was an average deficit of 450 kcal/day in the reported intakes.[17]

All these issues were re-evaluated in a large analysis by Tracy Burrows and colleagues from the University of Newcastle, NSW, Australia of research studies covering in total more than 6,000 people in whom reported energy intake (diaries) was compared with total energy expenditure, measured using the doubly labelled water method described in the previous chapter. Given the energy balance model, on average these two should match – or, if anything, given that on the whole people are gaining weight, intake might be a little bigger than expenditure. But almost universally reported energy intake was less than measured energy expenditure, and not just by a few per cent – typically by 20–30 per cent. Among the studies analysed were several that included 'a technology component', such as the use of a smart phone or a wearable camera. This made little difference to accuracy of reporting. Even more relevant to the present discussion, they noted that under-reporting of energy intake was seen to a greater degree in studies of adults with overweight or obesity compared to adults of normal weight.[18] We shall see again in chapters 6 and 7 how this issue has confounded our understanding of human energy balance, and particularly in the context of obesity, for decades, and how these misunderstandings still persist.

Energy balance – why we are so easily misled

In three chapters, including a lot of science, I hope to have shown you why I think the concept of energy balance is so problematic: why it is so easy for people, even the supposedly well informed, to cast doubts upon its validity. The problem, in essence, is this. There are two sides to the energy balance equation. On the outgoing side, scientists have methods for measuring energy expenditure with great precision, whether the subject be confined in a laboratory or, nowadays, with the advent of the doubly labelled water method, going about his or her daily business. But the input side is much more problematic. Even scientists who know about this will still, essentially, ask people what they eat. Indeed, that's how government statistics are gathered. And yet we can say for certain that even the most apparently sophisticated techniques – for example, supplementing food diaries with photographs of food – can be seriously misleading. (In later chapters we will see how this has really distorted views of human energy balance for far too long.) And for the majority of us, we base our judgements about our own, and other people's, energy balance, not from knowing anything about our or their energy expenditure, but on snapshots of eating behaviour. When I chat to my jogging friends, I don't ask them how much energy they expended overnight. I ask what they eat. When I sit with my colleague Fredrik in a remote hotel, he doesn't look at me, judge how much heat I am giving off, and comment on my metabolism: he looks at what I am eating and makes judgements from that, despite knowing that this can be seriously misleading as regards my usual daily life. When someone asks me why their metabolism is 'so slow', it's not that they have in any way set out to measure it: it's based on what they think they eat compared with other people they know. And, to be blunt, both those estimates are likely to be not much better than random numbers.

My own firm belief in the principle that 'a calorie is a calorie', and that energy balance is the overriding principle that governs our weight, comes from my research in human metabolism in different situations, some of them quite extreme, over many decades. When we examine just how we derive energy from the nutrients we eat, we see that all nutrients enter one single pathway for oxidation and liberation of their energy; and that the body has finely tuned mechanisms that sense what nutrients are around, and adjust what our cells need to do with them. To appreciate that, we need a little excursion into metabolic biochemistry.

4

The black box of metabolism

Why a black box? The physiologists of the eighteenth and nineteenth centuries studied animal growth, mainly farm animals, by measuring what they fed the animal, noting how it grew, and collecting and measuring what came out of the back end. What happened in between was to them a 'black box'. Now we call it 'intermediary metabolism'. Scientists began to understand it from around the middle of the nineteenth century, but new advances are happening all the time – several during my lifetime in research.

We are all solar powered

Oxford is surrounded by farmland. It's early summer as I write this, the crops are growing nicely after a wet spring, and now the sun is shining on them. It takes even a supposed expert in metabolism a bit of reflection to imagine that some of that energy coming to our fields from the sun might later in the year be powering me along as I jog or cycle.

We're going to discuss metabolism, but with a particular

emphasis on energy, which, after all, is the subject of this book.* Energy is a difficult concept. Scientists would define it as 'the capacity to do work', which is fine until you ask what exactly 'work' means. After a quick look at the energy coming to earth as sunlight, we'll deal mainly with chemical energy, and also heat, with a bit of physical work (moving muscles) thrown in. Different forms of energy can be inter-converted, and the laws of thermodynamics state that the total amount of energy in a system doesn't change. That's the basis of the idea of energy balance that is central to this book.

Chemical energy is the energy stored in the bonds between atoms when they join together to make molecules (groups of atoms joined to one another by chemical bonds). The energy can be released when the bonds are split apart – this is what we call a chemical reaction. Usually new bonds are then formed. To illustrate this, imagine some hydrogen gas and some oxygen gas mixing. Nothing will happen until a small amount of energy is put into the system (for example, a match): this energy simply starts the process, allowing the atoms to rearrange. Both hydrogen and oxygen exist as mole-cules with two identical atoms (represented H_2 and O_2); they react like this:

$$2H_2 + O_2 \longrightarrow 2H_2O + heat$$

This means that two molecules of hydrogen react with one of oxygen to produce two molecules of water, with release of heat. This heat comes from the bonds between the atoms in

---

* Of necessity, this will be a selective and abbreviated account of metab-olism. My student textbook, *Human Metabolism* (written with Rhys Evans), has 380 pages. My shorter primer on metabolism, *Understanding Human Metabolism*, will give you more information if you want to follow up any of this.

the molecules of hydrogen and oxygen. Water is a more stable molecule and its chemical bonds have less energy, so there is now energy to spare, which is released as heat.

We can also make this reaction go the other way, producing hydrogen and oxygen from water, but then we need to put in energy – this is the basis of the generation of hydrogen that some people believe will be the fuel of the future, made from water using, for example, electrical energy generated in turn from wind or sunlight.

We couldn't live without plants

You might consider yourself a meat eater but, nevertheless, you couldn't live without plants. Even if you don't eat plants yourself (which is difficult to imagine for a human – but it would be true, for example, for a cat), you are eating the meat of something (such as a cow – or a mouse if you are a cat) that has, in turn, eaten plants in order to grow. And that's where we get our energy.

Plants use the energy of sunlight to make a chemical reaction happen. That chemical reaction is the splitting up of a molecule of water (using light energy), releasing oxygen (the origin of the oxygen in our atmosphere, without which we couldn't live) and hydrogen atoms, which are used to drive the build-up of more complex molecules.

Living beings are made of molecules made from carbon, hydrogen, oxygen, nitrogen and a few other elements. Carbon atoms provide the skeleton for almost all molecules involved in life, called 'organic' molecules. Carbon dioxide, CO_2, the simplest, is the starting point for the building up of more complex molecules. Molecules of common sugars contain six atoms of carbon, usually arranged in a ring shape. Fatty acids, the building blocks of the fats we eat and store in our body, typically have a chain of sixteen, eighteen or more carbon atoms in their molecules. Amino acids, the building blocks of proteins, have anything from two to eleven carbon atoms. To these carbon atoms, arranged in chains or rings, are attached other atoms such as hydrogen, oxygen and nitrogen. Plants can make these more complex molecules from carbon dioxide, using the energy and the hydrogen released from water and sunlight – that is the process called photosynthesis. Animals can't do this: hence, we rely on plants.

Energy is used in building up these complex molecules. The energy is then stored in the molecule: that's chemical energy. Typically, that energy is released again by breaking apart the molecules with oxygen. This is the process called oxidation. Plant material will burn – its molecules will combine with the oxygen in the air. (Just as I mentioned for oxygen and hydrogen, a little input of energy – such as from a match – is needed to start the reaction going.) And energy is released – we feel the heat from a bonfire. But the process also goes on in a more controlled way inside our cells, as we saw in Chapter 1.

Just in passing, I might also have written, 'We couldn't live without bacteria.' Plants carry out the conversion of carbon dioxide, CO_2, from the atmosphere into carbon-containing chemicals that we need to live: we (all animals, in fact) cannot do that. It's called carbon fixation. But neither plants nor animals can 'fix' nitrogen, N_2, from the atmosphere to make amino acids and proteins. And yet, the web of life depends on amino acids. That reaction, taking N_2 from the air and making organic compounds, called nitrogen fixation, is a property of certain bacteria. Some of these bacteria live in association with plant roots, especially plants of the pea family. Amino acids can then be taken up by the plants – and, eventually, by us. If you imagine the great muscled bulk of an ox, that protein has come from the grass it eats, and that in turn has come from bacteria in the soil.* I think it's a strong argument for looking after our environment – but, I must say, it's not directly relevant to our present discussion.

The fuels of life

We've already met the three nutrients that provide almost all our energy: carbohydrates, fats and proteins. Each of these consists of large molecules – storing a lot of energy – built up from smaller units.

Sugars are the building blocks of carbohydrates. There are many sugars, such as glucose (the most common in our metabolism), named after the sweetness of grapes, fructose or fruit sugar, and galactose, named after milk in which it is found. Each of these has six carbon atoms in its molecules. These 'simple sugars' can join together. A larger molecule, made of one molecule each of glucose and fructose, is then called a disaccharide ('two sugars'), in this case sucrose or table sugar. Glucose and galactose combine to make the disaccharide lactose, the sugar found in milk. Disaccharides are common in our food supply.

It doesn't stop there. Glucose molecules can join in long chains, up to perhaps a few thousand. This is starch, found in plants. For the plant cells, it's easier to store these large molecules than many smaller ones. (There are different forms of starch: the chains of glucose molecules may be straight or have branches.) When we eat plant starches, they are broken down in our digestive system to release the individual glucose molecules, which can then enter our bloodstream through the

---

* Except that modern fertilisers used by farmers include nitrogen that has been 'fixed' from the air in an industrial process – one that uses energy and releases carbon dioxide into the atmosphere, a very environmentally unfriendly process.

cells of the intestinal walls. But we can also make starch! The animal form, glycogen, we store in our liver and our muscle cells (with small amounts in other tissues, including the brain). Glycogen consists of branched chains of glucose molecules, attached centrally to a protein, and forming a 'fuzzy ball', which means that there are lots of ends from which we can break off individual glucose molecules to use for energy.

A characteristic of carbohydrates is that they consist of molecules made of carbon, hydrogen and oxygen. The presence of hydrogen and oxygen makes them a little bit similar to water (H_2O), and they can all mix with water, or even dissolve in it. (All simple sugars will do that. Glycogen, like the cellulose in wallpaper paste, mixes with water, and hence is always stored in our cells with about three times its own weight of water – as we have seen, something that confounds many dieters.)

There are also things in our kitchen that we know don't mix with water – we call these 'fats' (chemists say 'lipids'). The fats in our kitchen – olive oil, vegetable oils such as sunflower and safflower, and animal fats like butter – are all made from fatty acids. Like sugars, there are a number of fatty acids, with names that tell you where they were first found: palmitic acid (first isolated from palm oil), whose molecules each have sixteen carbon atoms in a chain, stearic acid (eighteen carbons) from animal fats (after the Greek for tallow), oleic acid (also eighteen carbons) from olive oil. We don't have fatty acids as such in our kitchens. (I've tried eating fatty acids: they are horrible.) Three molecules of fatty acids combine with a chemical called glycerol or glycerine. Glycerol is technically an alcohol: it has three chemical groups (represented as -OH), one on each of its three carbon atoms, and each of which can attach to a fatty acid. That makes a larger molecule made of glycerol with three fatty acids attached, and this is called a triacylglycerol – or sometimes triglyceride. It sounds very chemical, but that's what we eat: olive oil, or any other kitchen fat, is made of triacylglycerols.

Stearic acid and oleic acids, mentioned above, each have eighteen carbon atoms in their molecules, but they differ. The molecules of stearic acid are formed on a chain of carbon atoms. All the spare chemical bonds are taken by hydrogen atoms. We say it's 'saturated' with hydrogen atoms and call it a 'saturated' fatty acid. Triacylglycerols made from it are called saturated fats. Because the chain of carbon atoms is straight and uncomplicated, molecules can pack together neatly side by side, and it is naturally rather solid (as in animal fats). In contrast, oleic acid's chain of eighteen carbon atoms is interrupted by two that each lack a hydrogen atom, and therefore join to each other with a 'double bond'. The molecule is not saturated with hydrogen, and fats made from it we call unsaturated. The double bond introduces a kink into the shape of the molecule, so the molecules can't pack closely together, and the fat tends to be more liquid – as in olive oil. Because there is one double bond, we call this monounsaturated. But there may be more double bonds. Linoleic acid, common in plant oils, has eighteen carbon atoms and two double bonds. Soya oil, corn oil and rapeseed oil all contain lots of linoleic acid, and are more liquid still than olive oil (olive oil will begin to solidify in the fridge). Linolenic acid, which is found, for example, in flax oil, has three double bonds in its eighteen-carbon chain, and makes fats that are yet more liquid. All these we call polyunsaturated. But – I hasten to add – from the point of view of energy, these differences are small. They may well be important for metabolic health, but the distinctions should not worry us when considering calorie balance.

Just as with carbohydrates, when we eat or drink fats containing triacylglycerols, the molecules are largely split apart in our digestive system, but they are recombined in the cells of the intestinal wall and enter the body again as triacylglycerols.

That sounds alarming! We've just seen that these things don't mix with water, but now they are in the bloodstream. Fortunately, we have evolved mechanisms for carrying these fats in the blood in minuscule droplets, technically an emulsion, in which proteins and other types of fat stabilise them. They are almost exactly the same as the fat droplets in milk, which are stabilised in the same way. In fact, after a fatty meal, our blood will turn milky, as the dietary fat enters and is carried around to where it needs to be stored, mainly in the specialised cells called 'adipocytes'. These cells make up body fat, or adipose tissue – the fat that lies under our skin, but also within our abdomen and in other tissues.

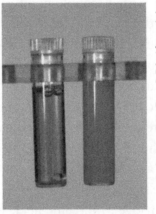

Credit: Frayn K.N., Evans R.D.[1] with permission

The plasma (the watery part of the blood) turns milky when we eat fat. Left, blood plasma taken after fasting overnight; on the right, a few hours after eating a fatty meal. The cloudiness is caused by the presence of dietary fat as an emulsion, like milk.

The role of amino acids in the body

There are twenty different amino acids that make up all our proteins, and more still that perform other functions. They can link one to another, making long chains of amino acids. The different amino acids have particular chemical characteristics, defining how they interact with other amino acids, and with the surrounding milieu, be it watery or fatty. When there are more than fifty amino acids in the chain, we call it a protein (shorter than that means that it is a peptide), and then the chain can begin to fold around, the different amino acids attracting or repelling each other; and that gives the whole molecule a specific three-dimensional shape.

Enzymes are proteins. Typically, an enzyme might have a few hundred amino acids in its chain. Its role is to bring about chemical reactions. It is, in chemical terms, a catalyst. Its particular molecular shape will enable it to interact, very specifically, with one or two smaller molecules – let's say a molecule of glucose and one of fructose – and provide the energy to start a reaction, just like applying the match to the bonfire. In that case, it might join the two sugars to make a molecule of sucrose. Enzymes bring about metabolism by changing chemicals, one into another, in organised pathways.

Of course, we eat enzymes and other proteins in plant and animal foods (in animals, most of the protein is in muscles). As with carbohydrates and fat, our digestive system will break apart the bonds linking the amino acids, and the amino acids can then enter our bloodstream to be taken up by cells and used to build our own proteins. Or, as with sugars and fats, they may be oxidised without being stored.

Metabolism in a nutshell

When we eat a meal that contains a mix of nutrients, as most meals do, these enter our digestive tract: the carbohydrates are broken down, and sugars (mainly glucose, from starch) enter our bloodstream; fats enter the bloodstream as triacylglycerols, and amino acids from dietary proteins also end up there.

(Babies can take up whole proteins, such as immunoglobulins, from their mother's milk, but this ability is lost during early development.)

Our tissues are primed to know what's about to arrive. Insulin (of which more shortly) is a major signal to say 'Stand by! Nutrients arriving!' Glucose will reach the liver cells, which take it up, and the enzymes that convert it to glycogen for storage will be activated. At the same time, the (different) enzymes that break down glycogen to liberate glucose are switched off. Fat arrives at our fat cells, adipocytes, and they are ready to take it up: triacylglycerols are temporarily broken down again to fatty acids, which enter the cells, and then they are recombined with glycerol to make triacylglycerols for storage. Again, at the same time, the enzymes that 'mobilise' our fat stores are suppressed. Once again, amino acids are a bit more complicated as the liver will grab some of them to make its own proteins and to make proteins that it sends out into the bloodstream; other amino acids will make their way to the muscles and other tissues. Those that are needed to make new proteins will enter that pathway (replacing old proteins that have been broken down), while others, especially those in excess, will enter the pathway of oxidation.

Now we are building up our energy stores: carbohydrate in the form of glycogen, fat in our fat cells. Each fat cell has one droplet of fat within it, taking up most of its volume, and expanding or contracting as new fat is taken up, or fat is mobilised. Proteins, again, are a little different. Every protein has a function, as an enzyme, as part of the system that makes muscles contract, as a transporter for substances into and out of cells, or as a structural component. There is no protein that is just there to store amino acids. That has consequences when we need to draw upon our energy stores. Glycogen and fat are used first, whereas protein is largely spared until the body has no other option.

As we saw in Chapter 2, carbohydrate in the form of glycogen is a small energy store. In contrast, the average of 25 kg of fat stored by participants in the Oxford BioBank holds enough energy for around 90 days. Why the big difference between our carbohydrate and our fat stores?

The answer is that glycogen is heavy for the energy it holds. As a carbohydrate, it will give us around 4 kcal for each gram. But, as it's always stored with water, this figure reduces to about 1 kcal for each gram of 'wet glycogen'. In contrast, fat can be stored with very little water. Each gram of fat stored will yield (allowing for the other things stored with it) 7–8 kcal. That makes a big difference when we need to carry around enough fuel to tide us through periods when food is unavailable. Perhaps if we were to evolve now, with constant food around, we'd have bodies that got rid of any excess – but we are lumbered with bodies that think famine might be just around the corner.

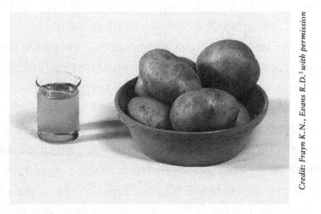

Credit: Frayn K.N., Evans R.D.[2] with permission

Illustration of the difference between fats and carbohydrates as energy stores. The picture shows 90 grams of olive oil and 1.05 kg (1,050 grams) of raw potatoes. Each would provide 800 kcal of energy. Raw potatoes contain water and carbohydrate in the same proportions as our glycogen stores. This shows the advantage of carrying our long-term fuel reserves as fat. It also emphasises the advantages of eating plenty of unrefined starchy food and cutting down on fat – you can feel full on much less energy.

Now for the 'calories out' side

After a typical meal, food is digested in our intestines and the nutrients enter the bloodstream over a period of a few hours. We've studied this in our research laboratories in Oxford and find that we don't return to a truly fasting state until around six hours after a meal. But after a sugary snack, it will be much quicker: there's less food to move along the intestines, digestion is quick and there will be a much faster rise and fall in the level of sugar in the bloodstream.

As those six hours pass, the body gradually changes from a state of storing excess nutrients into a state where it's ready to draw upon its energy reserves. It all happens seamlessly – I have written about it as one of the wonders of metabolism, that all these things happen without us having to think about it at all. And, of course, if we interrupt that period with a bout of physical activity, our muscles will need fuel, and we will start to draw upon our reserves more quickly.

We now need to look at the processes by which we derive energy from our stored fuels, concentrating initially upon carbohydrate and fat. In each case, there is a process called 'mobilisation', in which the stored fuel is broken down into its building blocks and released into the bloodstream. In the case of glycogen (starch) stored in the liver, this means that the enzymes that make glycogen from glucose gradually switch off, and those that break glucose units off from the glycogen molecules switch on. That glucose can flow out of the liver cells into the blood. (Glycogen stored in muscles is a little different. Similar enzymes can break it down to glucose, but that glucose cannot leave the muscle cells directly. Muscle glycogen is mainly a store for the muscles' own use.) Similarly, in our fat cells, enzymes that release fatty acids into the bloodstream switch on.

One feature of metabolism that is not always brought out, even in biochemistry textbooks, is that the different organs and tissues have different roles. It's something that my colleagues and I have stressed when teaching these aspects of metabolism to biochemistry students. (It's also a big focus of my student textbook.) I don't think it's surprising. We wouldn't expect a single factory to make everything, nor to use everything; we wouldn't expect a power station both to generate electricity and then to use it again. It's the same with metabolism: for example, only liver cells can release glucose in this way and only fat cells can release fatty acids into the blood.

There are also some differences in which tissues use fuels. The human brain is a big consumer of energy. But it cannot use our most abundant fuel, fat, directly. The brain is protected by a layer of cells that shield it from toxins, the blood–brain barrier, and fatty acids cannot cross this barrier. Glucose can, because of the presence of special proteins called 'transporters', which make holes for the glucose molecules to cross. Our muscles, including both the obvious ones in our arms, legs and trunk, and also the heart (a specialised muscle, which is using fuel all the time), are less picky: they will use glucose or fatty acids, according to availability.

Now I should mention amino acids. There is a tendency for our overall protein store to build up in the period after a meal, and to reduce again, liberating amino acids, as we begin fasting, but it's not nearly so pronounced as for carbohydrates and fats. (The major stimulus to build up proteins in our muscles is using them: exercise!) After meals, as dietary amino acids become readily available, the liver will readily use them for energy – by some accounts, they are the liver's biggest energy source. Muscles will oxidise some particular amino acids for energy.

Now imagine that the glucose and the fatty acids liberated

from our stores have been taken up into cells – we'll say muscle cells as an example – along with some amino acids. And we want to extract energy from them. As I mentioned earlier, this involves oxidising them – breaking them down by combination with oxygen (which we breathe in, and is then carried in the bloodstream to our tissues) to release energy.

Of course, it would be no use to us if these fuels were oxidised like a bonfire. We'd make lots of heat and nothing useful, so mechanisms have evolved that break each fuel down in small steps, trapping much of the energy that is released.

I am going to give a description of this aspect of metabolism that is, of necessity, a bit complex. I've made it as simple as I can, but if you want to skim over it, you will find the most important message of this chapter in the section following it on page 76.

ATP: the system for capturing energy

For all the fuels that give us energy, that energy is initially captured in a substance called adenosine triphosphate, or ATP. Every one of the 30 trillion or so cells in our body uses this system. But it's not just for us. ATP exists in all life forms. This system for capturing energy in ATP must have evolved at an extremely early stage in the development of life.

As its name suggests, molecules of ATP have three 'phosphate' groups. Ubiquitous in metabolism, phosphate groups are derived from phosphoric acid and confer an electrical charge on any molecule to which they attach. In ATP, the three 'phosphates' form a chain. Energy is needed to add them, especially the last one, which makes adenosine diphosphate (ADP), with two phosphate groups, into adenosine triphosphate (ATP). That energy – to make ATP from ADP – is the energy we're talking about, coming from our fuel stores. And once that's happened, ATP can deliver that energy to wherever in the cell it's required. For example, in muscles, it will deliver the energy needed by the proteins that make muscles contract. In the brain, it will drive the processes of electrical conduction that make us think.

ATP is made from ADP in a compartment of the cell called the mitochondrion. Most cells have many mitochondria (or mitochondrions). They are often called the powerhouses of the cell. When ATP is used to drive a process – muscle contraction is an example – it gives up its energy by splitting off the third phosphate group, becoming ADP. That ADP then goes back to the mitochondrion to be made back into ATP.

Nutrients are gradually broken down to liberate energy

How do we get ATP-energy from oxidation of glucose, fatty acids and amino acids? This is a key point for our story. They all enter a common pathway. They all feed into exactly the same system for trapping energy in ATP. Each of these nutrients is broken down by the small steps of metabolism into smaller molecules containing just two carbon atoms, in a form called acetyl-coenzyme A (or acetyl-CoA). (The smaller 'acetyl' component contains these two carbon atoms. Coenzyme A, always abbreviated CoA, is a larger component made from vitamin B5, pantothenic acid, and it is like a handle to pass the acetyl part around different metabolic pathways, without itself being altered.) One molecule of glucose, with six carbon atoms, makes two molecules of acetyl-CoA (two carbon atoms are lost as CO_2); one molecule of oleic acid, for example, with eighteen carbon atoms, will make nine molecules of acetyl-CoA; amino acids, as usual, differ, but many of them also break down to acetyl-CoA (some enter other pathways). And alcohol, called ethanol chemically, also goes to acetyl-CoA and joins the party.

Within the mitochondrion is a complex of enzymes that

break down acetyl-CoA into two molecules of CO_2. (The CoA part is recycled.) This mechanism is called the citric acid cycle, or often the Krebs cycle, after its discoverer, Hans Krebs. It is closely linked with another complex of enzymes that take the products of breakdown and transfer the energy into the enzyme called ATP synthase, which, as its name suggests, makes ATP from ADP and phosphate.

Why a calorie is a calorie

Complicated though the details might be, the whole is beautifully simple. There's one system, one final common pathway, by which we derive energy from all our fuels. Once they have become acetyl-CoA, there is no distinction between carbon atoms that came from glucose, fats, amino acids or, indeed, alcohol. This underlies my belief that 'a calorie is a calorie'. Metabolically, the different fuels are handled identically.

Ketone bodies

One aspect of the breakdown and oxidation of fatty acids will be relevant to us later. I noted that the brain cannot use fatty acids to fuel its large energy requirement. This could be seen as a problem during food deprivation, when we want to use our fat stores. But during starvation another pathway becomes important. When fatty acids are broken down in the liver, much of the two-carbon acetyl-CoA that is released will enter the citric acid cycle for oxidation. But some will enter another pathway, in which pairs of acetyl-CoA molecules will join to make a compound called acetoacetic acid, with four carbon atoms in its molecules. This is one of the compounds known (for historical reasons) as ketone bodies. The other major ketone body is 3-hydroxybutyric acid (made from acetoacetic acid by an enzyme), and there is a lessor one, acetone, which has only three carbons in its molecules and forms spontaneously from acetoacetic acid. These ketone bodies are made from fatty acids, but they are not lipids. They dissolve in water and can be taken up by the brain – and most other tissues – and used for fuel. In some heroic experiments on starving volunteers in the 1960s, blood samples were taken from the major blood vessels carrying blood to, and from, the brain, and showed that ketone bodies might provide two-thirds of the brain's energy requirements. Ketone body levels in blood are, essentially, a marker of the rate at which fatty acids are being used as a fuel.

High levels of ketone bodies in the blood are known as ketosis. This can be associated with beneficial health effects (for example, if it prolongs survival during starvation) or very bad health effects (in people with diabetes, when lack of insulin may cause ketone body levels to rise quickly). Somehow this bit of fundamental biochemistry has been adopted by proponents of diets, generally called 'keto diets', that involve restricting carbohydrate intake to the extent that the body goes into ketosis. In Chapter 10 we will come back to this and see whether, indeed, ketosis can lead the body to transgress the usual laws of physics.

Who's in charge here?

The above brief description skirts over a fundamental question. 'OK,' I hear you say, 'you said that enzymes switch on and switch off when food becomes available, or is running out: but who exactly told the enzymes to do that?' It's a good question. It's one that I have spent much of my research career investigating.

It brings us to the science called endocrinology – the study of hormones. Hormones are the 'who exactly?' Hormones are chemical signals that travel through the bloodstream conveying a message. Adrenaline is a hormone. It's released from the adrenal gland above each of our kidneys ('renal' means 'to do with the kidney'; hence the name).* When we feel stressed or threatened, the brain sends signals via nerves to the adrenal glands telling them to release adrenaline. Adrenaline (which is derived from an amino acid) travels in the blood. Many tissues make a protein called an 'adrenaline receptor'. (Actually, there's a big family of these, broadly divided into alpha- and beta-adrenoceptors.) The adrenaline receptor sits in the membrane surrounding the cell and has a shape that will specifically recognise adrenaline. Adrenaline comes along, binds to – or 'docks with' – the receptor, like a lock with a key, which then transmits a signal into the cell. Among other things, adrenaline will signal to the cell to switch on the relevant enzymes to start breaking down glycogen and, in the fat cell, breaking down stored fat. This releases fuels – glucose and fatty acids – into the bloodstream so that we have energy readily available to help us deal with the aggressor – or to run away. This is the fight or flight response, described by the American physiologist Walter Cannon in 1915. Adrenaline is also involved in mobilising fuels when we start to exercise.

Adrenaline, however, isn't involved in a major way in the changes brought about by feeding or fasting. This role is taken by two hormones that are released from the pancreas: insulin and glucagon. The pancreas sits just below the liver and its major role is to release digestive juices into the intestine. Within it are specialised groups of cells (called the 'islets of Langerhans', after their discoverer in 1869, Paul Langerhans) that produce hormones. These hormones are released into the bloodstream and first pass through the liver, where they

---

* In the USA, and some other countries, adrenaline is called epinephrine. And kidney doctors are called nephrologists.

have big effects. Insulin and glucagon are both small proteins. Insulin molecules have fifty-one amino acids in two chains, linked by chemical bonds. It is the hormone that signals a well-fed state and sends the body into storage mode. It is released from the islets when the concentration of glucose in the blood rises, a response that is augmented by fatty acids and amino acids. In liver cells, insulin will dock with a specific insulin receptor, which again sits in the outside membrane of the liver cell, and this will bring about changes within the cell. It will switch on the enzymes that make glycogen from glucose, and also switch off the enzymes that break down glycogen. The net result is that we use the glucose coming from the meal to rebuild our glycogen store. In addition, in muscles, insulin promotes the uptake of glucose from the blood. Then the glucose can be used as the immediate fuel for energy production and any excess stored as glycogen. At the same time, insulin is working on the fat cells. Here, similar to its role in liver cells, insulin strongly switches off the enzymes that mobilise our fat stores, and it activates the process by which fat cells take up dietary fat from the emulsion droplets that are in the blood after a meal. Insulin also has a general effect, stimulating the building up of proteins from spare amino acids. All in all, when insulin is released, the body preserves, and builds up, its fat stores; it preserves its proteins; and it switches into a 'glucose mode', using glucose and storing any spare as glycogen.

Glucagon, which I have mentioned for completeness, has more limited roles – or at least we think it does, perhaps because it's rather difficult to study. After it reaches the liver, very little of it is left to get into the rest of the bloodstream, and it's difficult to show changes in level by taking a blood sample from a vein in the arm, for example. In the liver, glucagon activates the enzymes that break down glycogen, so its role is opposite to that of insulin. It acts overnight to keep glycogen mobilisation going, but it probably has little role during a fed day. And despite the fact that fat cells have receptors for glucagon, it is now accepted that it doesn't have a role in fat mobilisation. Because of its role in glycogen metabolism, purified glucagon is used by people with type-1 diabetes (who lack insulin), when they have taken too much insulin by injection and their blood glucose level is getting dangerously low. A shot of glucagon (by injection) will quickly cause liver cells to break down glycogen and release glucose into the blood.

Some other hormones and their roles

There is a host of other hormones that are involved in metabolic events. The intestinal tract itself releases hormones that tell us when we need to eat and when we are full, that also tell the stomach walls to release acid when food is arriving, the pancreas to release its digestive juices into the intestine, and the intestines to move things along more quickly or more slowly. Then there are hormones that tell us about our body state: one of particular relevance is leptin, which tells us when we are accumulating too much body fat – or, more probably, warns us strongly when we are getting too thin. I will touch more upon these hormones in the next chapter.

I ought finally to mention thyroid hormone, a modified amino acid that is released at a fairly steady rate from the thyroid gland in the neck, and controls our general rate of metabolism – fast or slow. It seems to do this by acting in cells on the link between oxidation of acetyl-CoA in the citric acid cycle and generation of ATP – the step called 'coupling'. It may tend to 'uncouple' this process so that we oxidise fuels without generating so much ATP. Amazingly, more than a hundred years after its discovery, we still don't have a clear explanation for how thyroid hormone works. We'll look at that again in Chapter 6.

Coming back to calorie balance ...

When I moved to Oxford in the middle of my career, I was developing an interest in just how we, humans, store fat in our fat cells. That metabolic pathway was well worked out in small animals, but we really didn't know just what happened in ourselves. One feature of interest was this. In laboratory rats, the pathway by which we can make fatty acids from glucose had been worked out in the 1960s.[3] Essentially, glucose is broken down, as it would be for oxidation, into two-carbon units, acetyl-CoA. These molecules of acetyl-CoA can be added together, sequentially, to make a chain of carbon atoms: a fatty acid. It's a pathway called *de novo* lipogenesis (lipogenesis meaning creation of lipid, or fat; *de novo* meaning building up from scratch). There was (and still is, I might add) a common belief that eating carbohydrates would activate this pathway and so we would become fat. This pathway is stimulated, of course, by insulin – the storage hormone. I learned about this pathway as a biochemistry student. In our early married life, my wife, Theresa, and I avoided bread and potatoes because – as I would explain to her – these will make us fat because of the effect of insulin. I had long foreseen what the proponents of the carbohydrate-insulin model are now claiming.

I was wrong, though, and as I researched in this area, and read more, we changed our eating habits, worrying much more about dietary fat (which, as we will see in later chapters, can add calories to a meal without filling you up – as illustrated on page 71, 'Illustration of the difference between fats and carbohydrates as energy stores'). Why was this wrong? Firstly, we are not rats. Laboratory rats eat a low-fat, high-carbohydrate diet. They need this pathway of *de novo* lipogenesis to build up fat stores. We don't – we mostly eat enough fat to build up our fat stores as much as we need, if not more. 'Ah,' you may say, 'if I were only to eat carbohydrate, then, I couldn't add any fat.' (I note that this is the opposite view to the carbohydrate–insulin proponents.) But again, that's too simple. Insulin not only stimulates the pathways of laying down fat but also an equally strong effect is to prevent the mobilisation of what fat we do have. Switching off fat mobilisation is thought to be the metabolic process that is most sensitive to the effect of insulin – we've studied it by dripping insulin into volunteers' veins and have seen that it switches off fat mobilisation as fast as we can measure it. And we can't live on an entirely fat-free diet. Almost everything contains some fat. Indeed, we need certain fatty acids that we can't make ourselves in metabolism: these particular polyunsaturated fatty acids are known as essential fatty acids.

Instead, as we have shown over many years, the bulk of our fat stores are laid down by the fat cells taking up the dietary fat that circulates in the bloodstream after a meal (as in the illustration on page 68, 'The plasma (the watery part of the blood) turns milky when we eat fat'). It's an interesting process – it's been the focus of a lot of my research over many years – but it's a little complex to explain here, and not really relevant to our story.

That's not to say that humans don't have the metabolic pathway for making fats from sugars. It does exist, but its function – at least in those of us eating typical 'Western diets' – isn't to lay down fat. This has been shown in several experiments in which volunteers have eaten large amounts of carbohydrates and still they don't use this pathway to lay down fat except under exceptional circumstances – like being overfed (more than their energy requirements) with a carbohydrate-rich diet for a week or so (more on this in Chapter 9). But the importance of this metabolic pathway is something else, discovered in the 1970s. A key intermediate in the pathway of *de novo* lipogenesis, called malonyl-CoA (it's like acetyl-CoA, but the malonyl part has three carbon atoms), feeds back on the pathway for fatty-acid oxidation and suppresses it. It's a beautiful mechanism: carbohydrate intake suppresses fat oxidation; one fuel spares another. It's but one example of the way different fuels interact to ensure that our tissues have just what fuels they need, no more and no less.[4]

I'll sum up by coming back to calorie balance. When our body has an energy surplus – that is, more energy coming in than is needed for our energy expenditure – a symphony of mechanisms comes into play to store away the excess. We will refill our glycogen stores and put fat into our fat cells. Any long-term surplus increases this store of fat in our fat cells. Fat (triacylglycerol in fat cells) is the ultimate reservoir for excess energy. Much of this is coordinated by insulin.

These are the mechanisms that regulate our metabolism. But, as I've hinted, other mechanisms may affect just what we choose to eat, or not to eat. These mechanisms have been the subject of research for more than 100 years, although much of our understanding is very recent.

5

My trousers have shrunk! Outside and inside perceptions and the regulation of calorie balance

You may be reading this because you have issues with your weight. Perhaps weight is a bit like the family dog: some people will feel it behaves according to what we would wish; others will feel it has a mind of its own – it doesn't seem that you are in any way in control of what your weight (or your dog) gets up to. Certainly, when we looked at the problematic observations of energy balance in the army cadets studied by Edholm and colleagues in Chapter 3, we saw little evidence that energy balance or body weights were regulated in any predictable way, at least in the short term. In fact, human energy budgets often appear to vary widely in a rather random fashion, leading some expert nutritionists to argue that our energy demands are quite unpredictable.

Yet a lot of evidence points the other way. We know of many mechanisms that exist to help us regulate our energy balance, although these might always be overruled by external factors (such as highly desirable food).

In some people, energy balance is extraordinarily precise

When the University of Oxford introduced a course for medical students who had already studied some related discipline ('Graduate Entry Medicine'), I was given the task of teaching them nutrition and metabolism. They were, at first, a small group, and we had informal seminars and discussions rather than formal lectures. In general, their biological knowledge was stronger than their maths, so I could occupy a little time by asking them to do some simple calculations – like this one:

Many people don't change their weight much during adult life, some hardly at all. Let's imagine that a student, aged twenty, weighing 65 kg, might change energy intake and expenditure somewhat as his or her life progresses, and, at the age of forty, weighs 70 kg. I don't think that's unrealistic. The body weight has increased by 5 kg over twenty years. How closely has that person matched energy intake and energy expenditure?

Adipose tissue, where our fat is mostly stored, has cells (adipocytes) largely filled with fat, but with some cell fluid (cytoplasm), a nucleus and other components such as mitochondria. An approximate figure for adipose tissue energy storage is 7,200 kcal/kg. (It would be 9,000 kcal/kg if it were pure fat, based on the 'Atwater factor' (explained on page 34) of 9 kcal per gram.) Then this 5 kg increase in weight (assuming it to be mostly fat) represents an imbalance of 36,000 kcal (= 5 × 7,200) over twenty years, or, per year: 1,800 kcal (= 36,000/20). That's around 5 kcal/day. For someone eating three meals a day, each meal is matched – on average – to energy needs to within 1.6 kcal. On a typical energy intake of around 2,500 kcal/day, energy intake and expenditure have been matched to within 0.2 per cent. Over that time, we have eaten something like 6 tons of food. This seems quite remarkable. How is it achieved?

None of us could do that consciously. I have to say in all fairness that the calculation is rather over-simplified for reasons we'll come to later, but the conclusion that energy intake and energy expenditure may, in some people, be matched with an astonishing degree of precision still holds. To look at it another way, our calories 'in' and 'out' must be balanced very precisely if we wish to keep our weight steady.

There are differences in how this precision might be interpreted, however. There are three main explanations for the ability of some people to maintain a very constant body weight. Looking at these may also help us to see the reasons why others find it so difficult.

External cues and energy balance

One idea about regulation of energy balance, in so far as it exists, is that it's largely down to external cues. The late John Garrow, author of the textbook *Energy Balance and Obesity in Man*, was a physician with expertise in treating obese patients, and a researcher in obesity. When I got to know him, he was working at the UK Medical Research Council's Clinical Research Centre in north London. He wrote much common sense about the reasons people become obese, and how to treat the condition. But he was also an observer of his own habits – as I have mentioned, like many others involved in the obesity field. In fact, he proposed that all those working on body-weight regulation should record their own experiences, as this would provide a vast database; he suggested setting up the SEOOAH, the Society for Enquiry into One's Own Alimentary Habits. I am not aware that it ever took off. Garrow carried out, and recorded, a number of experiments on himself, as he said 'poorly conceived and badly controlled', but nevertheless illustrative. His weight tended to be constant at about 76 kg, so he regarded this as his 'naturally preferred' weight. (We will see later that the idea of a natural 'set point' for one's body weight is widespread among obesity scientists.) He then deliberately changed his weight. Initially he over-ate to drive his weight up to about 80 kg, assuming that it would then return to his 'normal' 76 kg. He had someone else weigh him and record his weight so that he didn't know the result, and indeed his weight dropped a little, but not back to 76 kg. Only when he knew the readings did his weight return to 76 kg. Later, for different experimental purposes, he deliberately lost 5–6 kg in weight, expecting that he would then return to his 'preferred' weight. Again, he had someone else weigh him without telling him the readings. In fact, his weight returned rapidly to 76 kg and then kept going up, until, as Garrow says in writing about these experiments, 'I was unable to ignore the fact that my clothes were unusually tight, so I could not maintain the 'blind' condition' (that is, not knowing his weight). Garrow came to believe, in other words, that any constancy that is observed in adult human body weight is down to external cues – the reading on the bathroom scales, or the tightness of the trouser belt.[1]

In a letter John Garrow wrote to me dated March 2004, he discusses a statement made by the Edinburgh physiologist Reg Passmore, in the authoritative textbook *Human Nutrition and Dietetics*: 'Forty years ago, as an undergraduate, RP [presumably the author] had a tailcoat made for him ... He still wears the coat occasionally, and it still fits: ... [his] weight has never varied by more than 5 pounds [2.3 kg].' Garrow says in his letter to me: 'Passmore believed this to indicate "that food intake had a regulatory mechanism of great precision" ... I thought this was nonsense ... It seemed much more probable that the tailcoat WAS the regulatory mechanism of great precision: if he found that it did not fit, he was (being a Scot like myself) much more likely to adjust his food intake than go and buy a new coat.'[2]

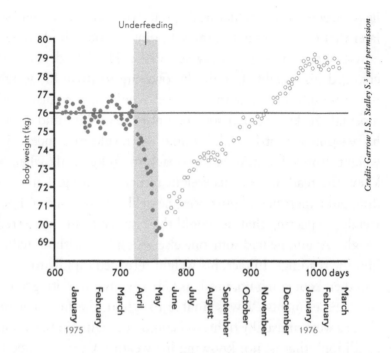

Credit: Garrow J.S., Stalley S.[3] with permission

John Garrow's self-experimentation. Garrow felt that his weight was naturally steady at around 76 kg. He lost weight deliberately, then without weighing himself, waited to see if his weight would return to 76 kg and stay there. (The open circles are his weight as recorded by an observer, who did not tell Garrow the result.) In fact, his weight continued to drift upwards until he realised that his trousers were too tight.

Garrow followed this up with a story from his obesity clinic. Patients came into the hospital's metabolic ward and stayed for three weeks, following a restricted diet, usually around 800 kcal/day. His PhD student, Penny Warwick, asked each patient at the end of their stay how much they thought their weight had changed. The patients, he says, 'wore rather baggy theatre tops and trousers while on the ward'. After the patients had given their verdict, they were handed their own clothes in which to go home, 'and they immediately revised their estimate of weight change to a much more accurate figure'.[4] This result, he added, strengthened his own belief that external cues are the prime sensors on which body-weight regulation depends.

I think it's difficult to argue with that. If you feel your weight now is not what you would like it to be, how do you sense that? Or if you feel it is creeping up, or down, how do you know? Is some signal within your body telling your brain that your fat stores are either a bit depleted, or a bit too replete? Or did you realise that your belt was not quite so comfortable as it used to be, or that the reading on your bathroom scales was gradually increasing (or decreasing)?

That, then, is one idea – that any constancy that we see in human body weight is down to external cues. Yet there has long been evidence for something more 'internal' than this.

Internal mechanisms to regulate energy intake

As early as the 1840s, it was recognised that people with brain injuries sometimes become obese.[5] In particular, this seemed true of damage in the area of the hypothalamus. The hypothalamus is a small (around 4 grams) – but very impor-tant – region on the underside of the brain. It is responsible for the integration of signals coming from the body, and the coordination of many of our physiological responses; for example, temperature regulation, thirst and, as we shall see, appetite. Just under the hypothalamus, and connected to it by a stalk, is the pituitary gland, responsible for secretion of hormones that regulate many aspects of bodily function, including thyroid function (which in turn regulates energy expenditure), sexual function, urine formation and stress responses via cortisol secretion from the adrenal glands. The phenomenon of obesity linked to hypothalamic damage was later named Fröhlich's syndrome, after Alfred Fröhlich, the Austrian neurologist who described it in 1901.

It's much easier to investigate brain function in laboratory animals than in humans. By the 1940s, it was possible to make extremely precise lesions at particular points of a rat's brain, by inserting a fine electrode while the animal was anaesthetised, and passing an electric current to destroy the local area. A.W. Hetherington in Chicago showed that the particular part of the hypothalamus that caused obesity when damaged was the ventromedial hypothalamus (VMH). The rats with VMH lesions ate much more than their unoperated-on companions, and hence gained weight: this was the site of regulation of energy intake (we might say appetite), although not energy expenditure.

Energy balance regulation: from conjoined twins to the discovery of leptin

In 1878 a young farming couple in Bohemia were expecting the birth of their second child. To their amazement, not just one but two babies were delivered, joined at the base of their backs. These conjoined sisters, the Blažek twins Rosa and Josepha, were the subject of intense media interest and medical attention. They remained conjoined throughout their 43-year lives. They could stand on two, three or four legs, and when one walked forwards, the other, of necessity, walked backwards. Not surprisingly, they were exhibited at shows and carnivals and acquired a manager, generating income for the twins and their parents. It is suggested that the manager was then responsible for Rosa conceiving a baby at the age of 32 years.[6] Our interest is in the fact that when Rosa breastfed her baby boy, Josepha also lactated. Since their blood circulations were joined, this pointed to a blood-borne factor controlling lactation – we would now recognise it as the 'love hormone': oxytocin.

There is a clear series of events linking these conjoined twins to the later discovery of the hormone leptin, a key component of the system that controls appetite in mammals, including rodents and people. Much of the experimentation involved studies on rats and mice, and since this is a book about human energy balance, I won't go into detail except to show the thread.

The case of the conjoined twins, while not itself directly relevant to our investigation of energy balance, was cited by the physiologist G.R. Hervey (always known by his middle name, Romaine) as the inspiration for his work with VMH-lesioned rats, at the University of Cambridge in the 1950s.[7] Hervey was a medical student in Cambridge during the Second World War who, coincidentally, answered an appeal in 1942 to volunteer for experiments led by Robert McCance, head of the Department of Experimental Medicine – McCance was one of the investigators we met in Chapter 3, well known for his nutritional work with Elsie Widdowson. The work involved immersion in cold water to try to improve the survival of airmen who had crashed in the sea, and one practical outcome was a covered inflatable life raft. Hervey retained an interest in naval matters throughout his career, alongside his work on obesity.[8]

After reading about the Bohemian twins, Hervey joined the circulatory systems of two rats, a technique called parabiosis. He found that if he made a VMH lesion in one of the rats, the animal subjected to the lesion ate voraciously and gained weight (as was the case for a single rat), while the other rat, not lesioned but sharing the same blood supply, ate less than before, became thin, and sometimes died in an emaciated state.[9] Hervey deduced that some signal in the lesioned, over-eating rat was then, via the linked bloodstreams, signalling to the brain of the unlesioned rat and causing it to eat less. He thought that the 'signal' probably showed how much fat the animal had stored. The lesioned rat could not respond to the signal, as its hypothalamus (the part of the brain that controls eating) was damaged. Hervey had correctly identified the workings of a major system of appetite regulation. I met Hervey some years later, when he worked at the University of Leeds; we corresponded about energy balance in obesity. We shall look at that in Chapter 7.

Doug Coleman, at the Jackson Laboratory in Bar Harbor, Maine, was inspired by reading Hervey's work to do parabiosis experiments, as Hervey had done with the hypothalamic-lesioned rats.[10] Coleman used as a model two strains of mice discovered in that laboratory, which had a natural tendency to overeat and become obese, one of them (with a slightly different genetic background) also to develop diabetes. Coleman linked the circulations of different combinations of these mice, and deduced that one strain, known as *ob/ob** (*ob* standing for 'obese'), could not make a signal to reduce food intake when the body's fat store grew, and hence kept eating; this signal was presumably the one Hervey had suggested. The other strain, *db/db* (for 'diabetes'), on the other hand, could not respond to the signal, although it could make it, and so equally kept eating – like Hervey's VMH-lesioned rats.[11] These findings were amazingly prescient. It would be more than twenty years before the signal was identified, but now there was a clear target: the gene called *ob*† that presumably held the clue to the mysterious signal, and perhaps the key to regulating appetite.

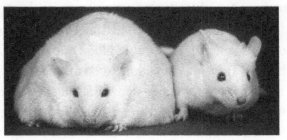

Credit: Wikipedia

An *ob/ob* mouse and a lean mouse for comparison.

---

* It's important to remember that the animal has two copies of each chromosome (one from each parent): only mice carrying the mutation on both their chromosomes became obese, so they were known as *ob/ob* mice. The same was true of the obese/diabetic *db/db* mice.

† Note that the gene is called '*ob*' or 'obese', but normally its function is to keep the animal lean. It's a mutation in this gene that leads to obesity.

The discovery of leptin, the 'fat hormone'

In 1994 Zhang and colleagues, from the research group of Jeffrey Friedman at the Howard Hughes Medical Institute and Rockefeller University in New York, used 'positional cloning' to find the gene in mice, mapping the position of the *ob* mutation on mouse chromosome 6 in finer and finer detail. They reported in *Nature* that the gene harbouring the *ob* mutation appeared to code for a 'secreted protein', a protein that might carry a signal – in other words, a hormone. They then looked to see in which tissue this gene was expressed – where the protein that it encoded was made. The answer was adipose tissue, the tissue where we, and the mice, store fat.[12] This is a signal made in adipose tissue. It signals to the brain to say, effectively, 'enough is enough'. (The more fat, the more signal is produced.) Friedman named it 'leptin', from the Greek *leptos* for 'thin'. The system does not work in the *ob/ob* mouse because the gene is mutated, and the mice cannot produce functional leptin. Nor does it work in the *db/db* mouse because, as Coleman had predicted, the receptor for that hormone in the hypothalamus is mutated, and the mouse cannot respond to the signal. This work from Friedman's laboratory, incidentally, changed our views of endocrinology: here was a hormone, leptin, produced not in one of the classical hormone-producing glands but in a tissue most people had previously thought was a rather inert store for surplus energy.

In the same paper from the Friedman group in *Nature*, the scientists looked for, and found, a similar gene in humans, and noted that the sequence of amino acids in mouse and human leptins was very similar (84 per cent identical), implying a protein with a very important biological function in mammals. For their joint parts in this important discovery, Doug Coleman and Jeff Friedman were awarded the 2010 Albert

Lasker Award for Basic Medical Research, regarded as second in prestige only to the Nobel Prize.

The discovery of leptin marked the beginning of a remarkable period of activity. Once the sequence of amino acids in the hormone leptin was known, it was possible to make it in the laboratory. When this synthetic leptin was injected into *ob/ob* mice, they became thinner. But when leptin was injected into *db/db* mice, there was no effect – the receptor was mutated, so they could not respond, however much leptin they received. In 1996, the gene for the leptin receptor, the gene known as *db* in mice, was identified, and again a human version of the leptin receptor was found, with close similarity to that of the mouse.

An obvious question would then be whether obese people, like the *ob/ob* mouse, are unable to produce leptin. The answer to that came soon after the discovery of leptin. By 1996, Robert Considine at Thomas Jefferson University, Philadelphia, had developed a method to measure the concentration of leptin in blood and made measurements in lean and obese people. The answer was clear: obese people in general have high, not low, leptin concentrations. This is to be expected: as their adipose tissue expands, so they produce more leptin. But it rules out a defect in leptin production as a common cause of obesity. Considine and colleagues also showed that, as obese people lost weight on an 800 kcal/day diet, so the concentration of leptin in their blood fell.[13] The system behaves in humans as we would expect it to, from the mouse studies.

There was enormous interest from the pharmaceutical companies. Would injections of leptin, the signal to reduce eating, or perhaps a drug that mimicked its action, be the 'cure' for obesity? Leptin is made in the laboratory, like human insulin, by recombinant DNA techniques. In the case of insulin, the DNA of the gene for insulin has been introduced into bacteria, and these bacteria can then be grown in large fermentation tanks. Human insulin (at least, a protein with exactly the same structure as human insulin) is released into the fermentation medium and can be purified for injection by people with type-1 diabetes. The same was done with leptin by the American biotech firm Amgen, who bought the rights to the gene for $20 million.[14] In 1999 Steven Heymsfield, a well-known researcher in the field of body composition and obesity at St Luke's-Roosevelt Hospital, New York, together with colleagues from Amgen, published the first results of a randomised, controlled study of leptin injections in seventy-three obese men and women. There was, on average, weight loss of several kilos in the obese volunteers after twenty-four weeks of treatment, most of which was body fat: but the weight loss was extremely variable, with some people not responding at all. A comment in *Science* summed this up as 'Leptin not impressive in clinical trial'.[15] Perhaps this was not surprising, albeit disappointing. After all, we knew by then that most obese patients already had elevated blood levels of leptin. Adding some more did not make much difference. There is now a belief in a state of 'leptin resistance', akin to 'insulin resistance'. Further trials have followed, some with modified versions of leptin, but as yet none has produced useful results.[16] There remains, though, the possibility of a sub-group of leptin-deficient obese people who might benefit.[17]

It would, however, be a mistake to think that leptin is irrelevant to human body-weight control. Stephen O'Rahilly at Addenbrooke's Hospital, Cambridge, had for some time been collecting details of patients who showed marked obesity from childhood, the 'Genetics of Obesity Study' or GOOS cohort. In 1997 O'Rahilly and colleagues published in *Nature* a paper describing two cousins, a boy and a girl, who had exhibited severe, intractable obesity from soon after birth. When the researchers tried to measure leptin concentrations in blood samples, they found none. They then looked at the gene for leptin, and in both children found a mutation (the same mutation) that would make leptin inactive. These children were the human equivalent of the *ob/ob* mouse.[18]

Since that time, a good handful of people around the world have been reported with this condition. And a few have been found with mutations in the leptin receptor, akin to the *db/db* mouse. It is important to note that this is an extremely rare condition, and nothing to do with 'common' obesity. Remember that, as I pointed out for the *ob/ob* mouse, the mutation must be present in both copies of the leptin gene (one on the chromosome from each parent) for these effects to appear. Mutations in the leptin gene are extremely rare, so this would be almost impossible in the general population: the cousins in the O'Rahilly group study were offspring of a consanguineous family, with marriage between close relatives, so that the mutation could be carried down the generations and then two copies come together in a subsequent generation.

Stephen O'Rahilly and his colleague Sadaf Farooqi, both physicians as well as scientists, have taken a strong clinical interest in these children. Given that human leptin was available, they worked with the Amgen scientists and gave the children injections of leptin. The results of this human experiment have been astounding, the leptin-deficient children returning to relatively normal weights.[19] There are now several reports in the literature of the success of leptin treatment in people with this deficiency, including adults. A family of leptin-deficient adults from Turkey were treated in the USA for eighteen months with synthetic human leptin, with remarkable normalisation of their body weight. But, sadly, those patients with mutations in the leptin receptor remain untreatable by leptin injection. Leptin has also proved to be a helpful treatment for the small group of patients who, because of a genetic mutation, lack normal amounts of adipose tissue:

hence they also (largely) lack leptin. Their metabolic problems are normalised to some extent with leptin treatment.

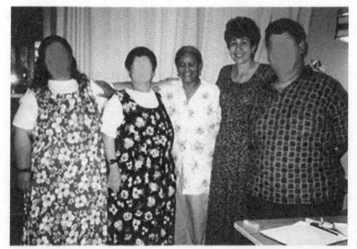
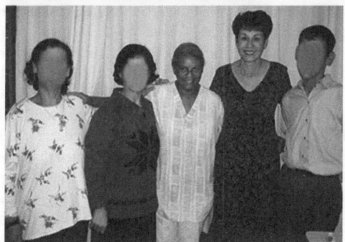

Credit: From Licinio J., Caglayan S., Ozata M. et al[20] with permission

Treatment of a family with leptin deficiency with synthetic leptin. Three related patients who lack leptin were treated with synthetic leptin for eighteen months. Their average BMI dropped from 51 to 27 kg/m^2. In the picture, two research nurses (centre and next right) are also shown for comparison; their weights were stable.

Our view of the role of leptin in human physiology has shifted as a result of these observations. Lack of leptin is an extremely powerful signal. Its main characteristic is an intense drive to eat. But the high leptin signal in obese people seems rather ineffective. Leptin in humans seems to have the role of protecting us against starvation: when body fat is lost, the leptin level in blood falls, and that brings about hunger. It's much less clear that high levels of leptin, as seen in most people with obesity, are doing much to restrain appetite.

It's in my genes

There is a clear inherited tendency to high body weight. Obesity runs in families. It used to be said that what ran in families was not the genes so much as the frying pan – that styles of cooking and eating were handed down in families, and this might have nothing to do with genetics. There must be truth in this argument, yet we now know that genes do have a large influence on human energy balance. Pioneering studies in the 1980s by the American physician Albert ('Mickey') Stunkard on Danish and Swedish identical twins adopted at birth and reared apart showed that, as adults, their body weight resembled their birth parents' rather than their adoptive parents' body weight. It is now accepted that around half the variation in weight among adults is down to genetics (estimates range from 40 to 70 per cent).[21]

Geneticists looking at what genes are involved in obesity have considerably increased our understanding of the regulation of energy balance in humans, sometimes building on research in experimental animals. There are two major approaches to finding genes responsible for medical conditions. One is to search for mutations in genes that one might expect to be involved, as was done for leptin deficiency. The other is to take very large numbers of people, and search blindly for areas of DNA that seem to track with the condition – in this case, with body weight. The former is known as the 'candidate gene' approach, the latter as a Genome-Wide Association Study, GWAS.

Research on naturally obese rodents had identified a pathway within the brain that links the receiving of the leptin signal and the regulation of appetite. This centres on a hormone called melanocortin, which acts within the hypothalamus and works through a receptor known as the melanocortin receptor (MCR). There is a family of five types of melanocortin receptor, called MC1R to MC5R. The melanocortin receptor involved in appetite regulation is known as MC4R. Stephen O'Rahilly, Sadaf Farooqi, Giles Yeo and their collaborators in Cambridge have shown, among their cohort of people with severe, early onset obesity, that the most common individual genetic change affecting body weight in children is a mutation in the MC4R receptor (the human gene is called *MC4R*). This mutation is dominant – someone does not need two copies of the defective gene to show an effect. Around 2–5 per cent of severely obese children have this mutation, 1 per cent of severely obese adults, and 0.2 per cent of unselected individuals living in England.* Remember that this mutation was identified initially in children, in whom the effects may be particularly prominent – adults are open to many influences beyond their genetics. Not all mutations in the *MC4R* gene cause complete loss of function. The group in Cambridge have shown that the more severe the mutation (that is, the less function that the receptor has), the more people harbouring that mutation will eat when given a test meal from which they can eat as much as they like. The importance of this system for regulation of human energy balance is clear: it is part of the system in the brain by which leptin from the fat stores regulates our appetite.

Scientists have now identified a number of genes that (when

---

* The group in Cambridge have created a website devoted to the *MC4R* gene at https://www.mc4r.org.uk/.

mutated) can contribute to early onset obesity: the GOOS cohort website states that they 'have identified 15 different gene disorders that can cause severe obesity in childhood'.[22] It is not relevant to the theme of this book to list them all, but it is important to say that almost all are genes that act within the adipose tissue-hypothalamus-signalling pathway and relate to control of appetite. They help us to understand the pathways that normally operate.

This candidate-gene approach identifies genes that have relatively major effects on body weight (although, with the exception of a few dramatic cases such as complete leptin deficiency, these are never on their own the sole explanation for obesity). The GWAS approach, in contrast, seeks out genetic changes with a smaller individual effect on body weight. Investigators using this approach have recruited larger and larger panels of people to search for small genetic changes affecting body weight. The Genetic Investigation of Anthropometric Traits (GIANT) consortium used meta-analysis (combing data from many studies, comprising more than a third of a million individuals). Such studies have led to identification of several hundred genetic loci – positions on the DNA – that can influence body weight. But the influence of each may be very, very small. It was recently estimated that '97 loci have been identified as accounting [in total] for about 2.7% of variation in body mass index'.[23] In addition, these studies can be difficult to interpret, as very often the investigators cannot say what the function of the gene concerned is – if, indeed, a gene is identified. In many cases a position in the DNA is located but not necessarily even within a gene. Giles Yeo, a member of the team in Cambridge, has become a television personality of late in the programme *Trust Me, I'm a Doctor*, and also an author of popular science books. But Giles is also a serious geneticist. He has written, of GWAS results, that 'hits', as the signals are often called:

can appear anywhere in the genome, within, near or far away from any coding sequence [that is, from any gene]. Thus, a major challenge in the field has been to translate these statistical hits into real biological insight. The key question is which of these genes are responsible for the association with obesity, and what is the underlying mechanism?[24]

So far as the functions of the genes identified by GWAS are known, it is again overwhelmingly true that most seem to relate to appetite, although a few might be concerned with energy expenditure. There was much excitement a few years ago when the gene called *FTO* ('fat mass and obesity associated gene') was identified in a GWAS searching for genes associated with type-2 diabetes. On closer investigation, it was found that its link with diabetes was mediated solely through its effect on body weight. It is the gene with the strongest link to body-fat content of all those identified from GWAS studies. There are two common forms of the *FTO* gene, one of which predisposes to weight gain. Someone with two copies of the 'weight gain' form of *FTO* will be, on average, 3 kg heavier than someone with two copies of the 'lean' form of *FTO*. But that does not tell us the mechanism through which it acts. At one time *FTO* was thought to act in adipose tissue, perhaps speeding up burning of fat. But that idea has faded, and the current view is that the culprit may not even be *FTO* itself but other genes very close to it in our DNA.[25] All in all, we are a long way from understanding the genetic regulation of body weight in the general population.

A gut feeling

There is another system of regulation of food intake. Signals from the gastrointestinal tract also govern our hunger, or fullness. Specialised cells in the lining of the gut secrete hormones. Some of these regulate digestion; for example, secretin, the first hormone to be discovered, by the British physiologists (and brothers-in-law), William Bayliss and Ernest Starling, in 1902. (Starling also introduced the word 'hormone'.) Secretin is released from cells in the small intestinal wall in response to acidity within the intestine, as food arrives from the stomach. It stimulates the pancreas to produce digestive juices. Other 'gut hormones' affect the secretion of insulin from the pancreas, enhancing the effect of an elevated concentration of glucose in the bloodstream. One such hormone is called glucagon-like peptide 1, or GLP-1 (it is similar in structure to the hormone glucagon, which is released from the pancreas). Drugs related to GLP-1 (the hormone itself is unstable in blood, so has a short half-life) have changed the treatment of type-2 diabetes, helping the pancreas to produce more insulin. But it has also transpired that GLP-1 affects appetite, probably acting through nerves that signal to the centres involved in the regulatory mechanisms we have been looking at in the hypothalamus.[26] If it were not for detailed molecular work showing how this is brought about, I would have a slightly sceptical approach to this story.

Some years ago, colleagues in diabetes research in Oxford were playing with the idea of using GLP-1 for diabetes treatment. They recruited volunteers and, since GLP-1 is a protein hormone and must be injected, they set up infusions of GLP-1 directly into the bloodstream to see what happened to insulin secretion. The volunteers reacted very strongly – by feeling extremely nauseous, if not actually throwing up. Anyway, drugs related to the GLP-1 system are now looking very promising for the treatment of obesity, presumably acting through the hypothalamic mechanisms, although just perhaps making people feel a bit nauseous and hence not wanting to eat. The drug semaglutide is one that has made the transition from diabetes medicine to weight-loss drug, and found popularity among online influencers (marketed as Wegovy). This is but one of many gut-hormonal systems that may act on the regulation of intake of single meals. Another is the hormone ghrelin, released from the walls of the stomach when the stomach is empty, and causing hunger – it is often now called the 'hunger hormone', although interestingly it was discovered as a substance that stimulates the release of growth hormone (*gh-rel*ease becoming part of its name). This is just to illustrate that the body has many, many potential mechanisms for regulating what we eat in the short term.

Regulation of energy expenditure

We have concentrated so far upon mechanisms that regulate eating behaviour, or appetite – in other words, energy intake. It's worth stressing once again that much of the underlying science has emerged from studies on laboratory rodents, although human genetic studies confirm that similar mechanisms also operate inside us. How strong these internal signals are for most of us is a moot point. As I pointed out above, most of us become aware that we need to think about what we are eating – or what exercise we do – because we find our clothes no longer fit comfortably.

If the body is indeed trying to regulate energy balance, perhaps it would be equally feasible that what is regulated is energy expenditure. That is very clearly so, even if we do not always have the same detailed understanding of the mechanisms involved. I have come to feel that this side of the energy balance model might be more powerful than the internal signals regulating what we eat. I will cover the numerical side of these changes in energy expenditure in later chapters (chapters 6 and 10). But here's a summary.

It is very clear that if we cut down on what we eat, then an early response is that energy expenditure is reduced. This results partly because of the loss of body mass, but the effect is greater than that. This reduction in energy expenditure when someone eats less is, of course, one of the factors working against the aspiring dieter. We shall examine the implications of that further in Chapter 10.

Is the converse true? Yes, it is also clear that when someone increases their energy intake, energy expenditure will increase. Again, this reflects in part the increased body mass. Whether there is an effect beyond that is a controversial area. We will examine this in much more detail in later chapters, both in the context of obesity and of experiments with overfeeding – producing 'experimental obesity'. (This is why my little calculation at the beginning of the chapter is not quite correct.)

Therefore, energy expenditure does, indeed, change in the short term in response to changes in energy intake – yet another mechanism that may help to keep our weight trajectory steady.

Regulation of energy balance – we are not laboratory rats

Consider what has been learned since the recognition of hypothalamic lesions and their link to obesity in the nineteenth century. We now have a phenomenal amount of information on mechanisms that should tend to stabilise body weight – increasing hunger when weight (or more specifically our fat store) drops, and at the same time decreasing energy expenditure; and decreasing the desire to eat when our fat stores are swelling, along with an increase in energy expenditure. Although many of these mechanisms were worked out in detail in laboratory animals, we know that they exist also in humans, and we know from detailed genetic investigations that in extreme circumstances, such as the loss of one critical component, they can indeed affect human energy balance severely. But let us remember that most obese people have high levels of leptin in their bloodstreams. If we could but look inside the hypothalamus, we would almost certainly see those neurons firing that should reduce the desire to eat. And yet, as we all know, the incidence of obesity continues to increase. This is a very modern phenomenon. But then our lifestyles have changed almost beyond recognition in the past few decades – the period over which obesity has also increased, so how are we to interpret this? Is it that, indeed, there has been some change – like a chemical contaminant in the environment, as some would have us believe[27] – that has changed our relationship to energy balance, so that it's now time to drop the energy balance model and look instead for specific features of what we eat and drink? Or is it that cheap, plentiful, often flavour-enhanced foods, together with many opportunities to reduce physical work, simply overwhelm these primitive mechanisms that probably evolved primarily to help us avoid starvation in our hunter-gatherer days, or as early farmers? (But, I hasten to add, with clear genetic influences on how much we are able to resist such changes.) I hope my view is pretty clear. All this we will examine further in later chapters.

6

Why isn't my metabolism faster?

Some unfortunate people are just destined to struggle with their weight. Others don't have the same difficulty. We slim people are apparently blessed with an intrinsically fast rate of metabolism: we burn off our excess energy without laying it down in our fat stores. If I dare to let slip at a social occasion that I am a researcher into human metabolism, there are not many people who will not want to know why their metabolism is 'so slow'. (I think I have only once met someone who claimed to have a fast metabolism and needed to eat regularly. He was a cross-country skiing and mountain walking leader, which just may have had some bearing on the issue.)

This concept has widespread backing from reputable sources. In Chapter 1 I quoted from the websites of the University of Cambridge and of Harvard Medical School, describing how some people appear to be able to eat just what they like without gaining weight – indeed, the Harvard entry specifically mentions people who can eat ice cream and cake and yet remain slim.

We are not talking here about those who burn off lots of energy in exercise: elite runners and cyclists, for example, will eat enormous amounts compared with most of us, without gaining weight. But that's not how we see the concept of fast metabolism. Rather, the idea implies an intrinsically fast metabolism at rest, a high 'resting metabolic rate'. But what could that mean in biological terms? And how real is the existence of such people?

Fast metabolism certainly exists – in the clinic

We can gain some insight from medical cases of fast and slow metabolism. The clearest example is seen with disorders of the thyroid gland. The thyroid gland, located in the neck, combines the amino acid tyrosine with the element iodine to produce thyroid hormone.* A low level of thyroid hormone is commonly due to dietary iodine deficiency, whereas an excess is usually caused by a defect in the thyroid gland or the pituitary gland that controls it. Patients with thyroid-hormone deficiency feel cold and put on weight, whereas those with an excess may feel hot and find themselves losing weight – signs of slow and fast metabolism, respectively. But variations in thyroid hormone within the normal range don't seem to affect metabolism – it does not regulate specific pathways on an hour-to-hour basis like insulin, for example.

There are other examples of fast metabolism. Immediately after a severe injury, our body shuts things down: blood circulation to vital organs may decrease, glucose metabolism is reduced, and metabolism slows, a phase known as 'shock'. But starting a day or two later, there is a phase of increased

---

* There are two thyroid hormones, with three and four atoms of iodine per molecule, called triiodothyronine (T3) and thyroxine (T4) respectively. T3 is the active form. I shall refer to 'thyroid hormone' for simplicity.

energy expenditure, or 'hypermetabolism'. This increase –
which can be up to 30 per cent above normal – can last for
several weeks. In this phase the body starts breaking down
its own fabric, driven by a surge of hormones linked with
the fight-or-flight response, probably to liberate substances
needed for wound healing. There is often obvious wasting
of muscle, and this can be detected in the urine as an increase in the nitrogen-containing compound urea, showing
that amino acids are being used as a fuel. The same thing
is seen in people acutely ill with sepsis, a life-threatening
condition that happens when the immune system overreacts
to an infection and starts to damage the body's own tissues
and organs. I remember a case in Manchester when we were
measuring energy expenditure and assessing nutritional
requirements in injured patients admitted to the hospital's
accident and emergency department. Alan was a farmer, and
one of his cows had (he believed, deliberately) crushed him
against a barrier. His spleen was ruptured, and he developed
sepsis in his abdomen, and was clearly hypermetabolic. He
was saved by the surgical team looking after him who were
also experts in intravenous nutrition. They gave his body
the nutrients it needed to start building up healthy tissues
again.[1]

Although we are still not sure exactly what causes the
hypermetabolism in these cases, it is clearly different from
what's going on in people like my jogging friend Bobby who
appear to be able to eat anything and not put on weight. These
patients are not in a steady metabolic state, whereas Bobby is.

We need, therefore, to look for metabolic mechanisms that
could contribute to a fast metabolism in otherwise healthy
people. It's worth just considering what this would mean.
Again, we are not here looking at people who have fast metabolism because they are very active physically (we shall
consider how physical activity contributes to energy balance

in Chapter 8). We are looking for mechanisms that might waste energy – that is, burn up nutrients without doing useful work. This is, of course, in metabolic terms inefficient. An efficient metabolism would capture all the energy it possibly can from nutrients, so, more specifically, we are looking for mechanisms that will generate heat – a process known as thermogenesis.

A prime candidate has to do with adenosine triphosphate, ATP – the energy-carrying molecule found in all living cells.

Can the body 'waste' energy?

As we saw in Chapter 4, ATP is made in the mitochondria, distinct structures in our cells where nutrients – carbohydrates, fats and proteins – are oxidised to produce energy. The nutrients are broken down in metabolic pathways into smaller components, and ultimately to the compound acetyl-CoA, which delivers two carbon atoms into the citric acid (or Krebs) cycle in the mitochondria for ultimate oxidation, so releasing energy which can be captured by making ATP.

No step in a metabolic pathway is totally efficient – not all the energy can be captured, so each step liberates a little bit of heat as a by-product. 'Normal' metabolism liberates enough heat to keep most of us warm most of the time. During exercise, fuels are flowing through metabolic pathways faster than normal, and more heat is liberated, especially in the muscles, so we feel warmer – I am comfortable jogging in a T-shirt, whereas I need a jumper to be comfortable sitting at my computer. Metabolic pathways that lead to production of ATP all have steps that act as brakes to slow them down when the cell has plenty of ATP. In most tissues, therefore, ATP is created only as fast as it can be used, limiting heat production.

Brown fat

There is one specialised tissue in which the above is not true, however, called 'brown adipose tissue'.* Unlike the more abundant white adipose tissue where we store most of our fat, brown adipose tissue evolved specifically to generate heat to help maintain body temperature. It is found only in mammals, especially small species, including newborn humans.[2] The smaller the animal, the bigger the challenge it faces in maintaining its body temperature. By contrast, larger mammals – such as adult humans – have more need to lose heat than to make it. Animals that hibernate, including bears, also need brown fat. As they prepare to wake up, they activate it to warm them up from the low body temperatures of hibernation.

Brown adipose tissue cells have many mitochondria. In these mitochondria the process that oxidises nutrients is 'uncoupled' from the making of ATP. This happens because the cells make a protein called uncoupling protein, UCP, that short-circuits the normal linkage – the energy derived from oxidation is simply lost as heat without making ATP. All metabolic pathways can then run without check. It's like traffic backing up when the vehicles some way ahead are stopped from proceeding. As soon as a gate is opened that allows things to move at the front end, even if it's a side-gate into a field, everything can start to move again. Brown adipose tissue has the apparently wonderful property of burning off nutrients rather than storing them.

---

* Brown adipose tissue is distinctly browner than white adipose tissue. (In humans, white adipose tissue is yellowish owing to the presence of pigments such as carotenoids from carrots and other vegetables – these pigments are fat-soluble so accumulate in our fat stores.) Like red muscles (the 'dark meat' when you eat birds such as chicken or turkey), brown adipose tissue gets its colour from the presence of many mitochondria and their iron-rich pigments all involved in using oxygen.

For decades, there was a general opinion that, in humans, only newborns have significant amounts of brown fat: it was not thought to exist in adults. That view changed in the early 2000s with more widespread use of the medical imaging technique called 'positron emission tomography', PET. This uses short-lived metabolic tracers such as glucose labelled with a radioactive fluorine atom. Tumours can be seen in a PET scan because they consume glucose at a high rate, and radioactivity accumulates in them. In the 1990s, when this technique was still new, radiologists noticed that some of their scans seemed to show radioactivity hotspots around the neck area. But these did not look like tumours, as they were symmetrically placed, left and right sides mirroring each other. In 2002 it was suggested that these sites were not tumours, but brown adipose tissue.[3] Researchers have since taken biopsies of these sites and confirmed this view.[4]

We now know that brown adipose tissue can be found in adult humans, although not in everybody. It becomes more abundant with cold exposure: people who enjoy swimming in icy lakes have more than most, and it is found more often in the winter months (see illustration below). An international group of researchers, led from Maastricht in the Netherlands, studied volunteers before and after ten days of exposure to cold (15–16°C for six hours a day). Scans showed that the amount of brown adipose tissue increased by more than a third, and when the volunteers were cooled down in a water-filled suit, their metabolic rate increased more.[5] (Our metabolic rate will speed up a little when we are exposed to cold, probably because of increased muscle tone.[6] If we shiver, this will be considerable because it involves muscular movement.)

The role of brown adipose tissue, then, given its location, seems to be to ensure that the brain is kept warm in a cold environment. Several studies have shown that lean people have more brown adipose tissue than obese, although these are controversial; for example, the group based in Maastricht compared lean with overweight or obese men. They found similar amounts of brown adipose tissue (by volume), but in the lean it was more active in taking up the PET tracer.[7]

Credit: *Professor Mike Symonds, University of Nottingham, UK*

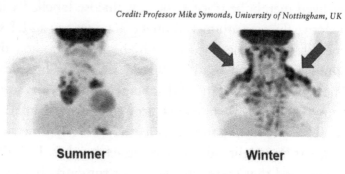

Summer   **Winter**

PET scans of one individual, showing that brown
fat is more prominent in winter (arrowed).

The big question remains: is there sufficient brown adipose tissue in adult humans to account for slow or fast metabolism – fatness and leanness? In other words, are there fortunate individuals who can eat all the cake they want because they happen to have a lot of brown adipose tissue? Most researchers now agree that this is unlikely. In a 2017 review, Eric Ravussin and Kara Marlatt at the Pennington Biomedical Research Center at Baton Rouge, Louisiana, concluded that, in adult humans, 'brown adipose tissue contributes a small amount to overall energy metabolism which is unlikely to cause weight loss'.[8] Since then, more detailed imaging studies indicate more brown adipose tissue than previously thought.[9] But still, in mice, brown adipose tissue represents 2–5 per cent of their body weight, whereas in human adults, the amount ranges from 0.1 to 0.5 per cent of body weight.[10] Its potential contribution to energy expenditure, even if maximally stimulated all the time, is a few per cent: certainly not enough to enable people to eat what they like without fear of weight gain. As Professor Mike Symonds, a brown-adipose-tissue expert, described to me, brown adipose tissue generates 300 times more heat (per gram) than any other tissue: it can't be *too* active or our brains would overheat.

That is not the end of the story, however. Under some conditions, such as cold exposure in small animals, normal white fat cells may begin to show features of brown fat cells: they start to make the uncoupling protein and they develop more mitochondria. These are now called 'beige' or 'brite' (brown-in-white) fat cells. Given that we all have much more white fat than brown, perhaps we can persuade our white fat to turn beige and burn off energy.

Although cold exposure in rats will increase the conversion of white adipocytes into beige, there is no convincing evidence that the same process happens in humans.[11] Therefore, although thermogenesis does increase when we are cold, this is not necessarily long-lasting. But there is still a belief that 'decreasing slightly our ambient temperatures or clothing compensations to cold, could be a less explored but more effective manner to promote better weight management control'.[12] Ice bathing or cold-water swimming could have even more effect. But, even if they could be shown to affect body weight, these seem unlikely to be sufficiently widely taken up to halt the worldwide increase in obesity.

More plausible is the hope that we may be able to develop a drug to increase our brown or beige fat. This could be a safe way to burn off excess energy and lose weight, unlike chemical uncoupling agents such as 2,4-dinitrophenol, which is promoted illegally on the internet for weight loss, but which can be fatal in humans. The idea is not implausible. Some people develop a tumour of the adrenal gland that leads them to make too much noradrenaline – the chemical that activates brown fat. They tend to lose weight. They also develop brown fat, showing that intense stimulation of white fat by noradrenaline can lead it to turn beige or brown. There are receptors that bring this about. Perhaps they could be targeted by a drug. But attempts so far to do this have been complicated by other features seen with these tumours, such as severely elevated blood pressure, which increases the risk of death from stroke or heart attack.[13] (It's a salutary reminder that all drug treatments come with adverse effects as well as the desired ones – perhaps especially in the field of body-weight regulation.)

A sufficiently selective drug has yet to be found. But there is another intriguing way in which the metabolism of those supposed fast metabolisers is possibly being stimulated – and that's overeating.

Eating to excess

Overeating? What does that have to do with staying slim? Not a lot directly, but much research over the years has looked at ways in which it increases energy expenditure.

Overeating – also called in this context 'overfeeding' – has been most closely studied in laboratory rodents. In a landmark study published in 1979, Mike Stock and Nancy Rothwell at Queen Elizabeth College, London, gave rats a choice of palatable high-fat foods such as 'chocolate chip cookies, salami, cheese, banana, marshmallows, milk chocolate, and peanut butter'. This became known as the 'cafeteria diet'. The rats gorged themselves, compared with other laboratory rats fed their usual boring low-fat hard pellets (called chow). To some of us, this was hardly a surprise. What was intriguing was that the rats coped with this excess better than humans. Despite eating nearly twice as much as the control rats, the cafeteria-fed rats put on only a small amount of extra weight. Instead, they increased the amount of brown fat between their shoulder blades and activated it to burn off much of the excess food – in other words, they developed a fast metabolism.[14]

Can humans do this too? The idea that some people can overeat but not put on weight has a long history. In 1902 the German physiologist Rudolf Neumann published results from experiments on himself. He found that he could overeat without a major change in weight, and first used the term '*luxuskonsumption*' to describe what he assumed was a switching-on of heat production to burn off excess energy.[*] Ethan Sims at the University of Vermont in 1973 described studies of prisoners overfed to produce what Sims called 'experimental obesity'. He found that they put on weight with overfeeding but needed 50 per cent more energy intake to maintain their elevated body weights. Undoubtedly these men would have increased their fat-free mass (that is, lean tissue) as well as their fat mass, which would have led them to need more energy, but we don't know enough about the experiment to tell whether there were mechanisms beyond that.[15]

In the early 1990s Patrick Pasquet and colleagues, based in Paris and at the Centre de Nutrition, Yaoundé, in the Republic of Cameroon, conducted a full audit of energy balance during overfeeding. They studied the traditional *Guru Walla* 'fattening session' among the Massa people of northern Cameroon. Over a period of nine weeks, young men will overeat two to three times their usual daily amount. Nine men volunteered to be part of the study. They were lean to begin with. During the overfeeding period they took in around an extra 4,800 kcal per day. Energy intake was 'corrected for energy in vomit', and digestible energy was 'corrected for losses in faeces and urine' – illustrating both the attention to detail taken by the experimenters and the

---

* The term '*luxus consumption*' is sometimes today used to refer just to excessive food intake.

difficulty of overfeeding at this level. The men gained an average of 17 kg: 11 kg of fat mass and 6 kg of fat-free mass. Total daily energy expenditure was measured along with resting energy expenditure and energy expenditure after meals and during exercise. Physical activity during the day was monitored with inventories and movement sensors worn by the participants. Unfortunately, given all that work – on the part of the participants as much as the experimenters – the results are somewhat confusing. Total daily energy expenditure did not change during the study (although there are technical reasons why the measurement technique may have underestimated this); but energy expenditure at rest, after meals and during physical activity all increased. The level of physical activity fell (probably the poor young men were spending too much time full up after eating to want to exercise). In all, the experimenters reckoned there had been about a 25 per cent increase in energy expenditure. Some of this would have reflected the gain of about 10 per cent of fat-free mass, some of it the metabolic costs of processing the additional food. But still, there was a remaining element of diet-induced heat generation or *luxuskonsumption*.[16]

Mike Stock, mentioned earlier, was a towering figure in obesity research for several decades. In 1999, just two years before he died at the age of 58 after a long battle with cancer,[17] he wrote a paper in which he reviewed these and other over-feeding studies.[18] Among other things, he looked at how 'efficient metabolism' (what we might call slow metabolism) depends on eating a well-balanced diet. For example, rats were fed a diet low in protein. As animals need protein in the growing phase in which laboratory rats are usually studied, they ate more of this diet than they otherwise would, trying to achieve the necessary protein intake. Rather than the rats getting fat, however, at least some of the extra energy (from carbohydrate and fat) was dissipated as heat – a form of diet-induced thermogenesis. But Stock also argued that this will occur when the diet has more protein than normal – there will be an excess of protein, which will be burnt off, so again there will be heat loss and metabolic inefficiency. He therefore suggested that there is an optimal balanced diet composition, which leads to the greatest metabolic efficiency; but 'imbalanced' diets, meaning diets with a low- or high-protein content, will lead to heat loss or fast metabolism. For rats, he showed that the optimal protein content of the diet supplied about 20 per cent of dietary energy.

Mike Stock's important contribution in that review paper was to collate data from human studies. These are all studies of deliberate overfeeding – that is, the volunteers were given more energy than they needed. Some were fed diets with high protein contents, some low. Mike identified a similar relationship between metabolic efficiency and dietary protein content, this time with the optimal protein content of the diet supplying about 12 per cent of dietary energy. But he also found great variability between people in how much extra heat they lost – perhaps, he speculated, this could be a test of how easily someone would gain weight, or otherwise, in daily life.

George Bray, an eminent obesity researcher at the Pennington Biomedical Research Center, has given his own perspective on such studies (appropriately, when giving the W.O. Atwater Memorial Lecture to the American Society for Nutrition). He discussed human overfeeding experiments, including Mike Stock's analysis. Bray had worked with Ethan Sims, who conducted the overfeeding experiments in prisoners. Later, Bray himself decided to try deliberate overeating, attempting to double his usual energy intake – which he couldn't manage, but he did manage to gain 10 kg. By measuring his own energy expenditure after this weight gain, he could test the idea that the diet-induced heat generation apparently observed in human overfeeding experiments represents the usual increase in energy expenditure that happens just after eating (called postprandial thermogenesis). He found no change. Nor did he find any change in metabolic efficiency measured during exercise. Bray and his colleagues then performed their own version of the overfeeding experiments, feeding men and women diets of low- and high-protein content. On the low-protein diet the volunteers indeed gained less weight, but this was because they failed to increase their fat-free (or lean) mass, accounting for their lower weight gain on that diet.[19]

For a final word on overfeeding, Eric Ravussin led a detailed study in thirty-five young people, mostly men – 'to our knowledge ... one of the largest and best controlled of studies conducted to date', according to the researchers, who published their results in 2019.[20] Each volunteer first took a dose of doubly labelled water (as explained on page 26) to measure their usual energy expenditure over two weeks. The experimenters then multiplied the daily energy expenditure of each subject by 1.4 to calculate the energy they would receive – that is, a 40 per cent increase above their requirements. All meals were then prepared in the research centre's own 'metabolic kitchen' and the volunteers came to the centre to eat their three meals each day under supervision. The protein content was 15 per cent of energy, close to what Mike Stock suggested was optimum for metabolic efficiency in adult humans. At the start and end of the eight-week overfeeding period, the volunteers spent twenty-four hours in a calorimetry chamber to measure daily energy expenditure as well as sleeping energy expenditure (using infrared sensors to detect when they were asleep).

The upshot of all this careful work was that the researchers found no evidence for diet-induced heat generation – that is, an increase in energy expenditure beyond that expected from any changes in fat-free mass. That's what we might have expected with this optimal protein-content diet. But there was an interesting follow-up observation. Most of the volunteers came back for a further assessment after six months. Those individuals who, during the overfeeding, had displayed less adaptation of energy expenditure tended to have retained more of the fat they had gained. Which brings us back to the question of whether some people naturally burn off a bit more of any excess energy intake than others.

To sum up, when people are deliberately overfed, energy expenditure increases. It does this mainly because the body lays down lean tissue as well as fat, and lean tissue is the component that expends energy. There is some evidence that certain people increase energy expenditure more than is accounted for by any increase in lean tissue, like the rats did in Stock and Rothwell's experiments, although this may depend on diet composition. Probably, as we saw in the previous section, humans just don't have enough brown adipose tissue to be like rats: perhaps a need to burn off excess energy hasn't been a driving force in our evolution. But others have argued that, even if there is a small effect of overfeeding, it is tiny in comparison with energy expenditure associated with physical activity.

Indeed, physical activity, although not necessarily in the form we might imagine it, forms the basis for one final mechanism that could lead to differences between people in their metabolic speed.

Muscular activity

Clearly, muscular activity is a way of dissipating energy. Nutrients need to be oxidised to make muscles contract, and this liberates heat as well as enabling us to do useful work externally such as moving from the ground floor to an office on a higher floor; we therefore lose energy from the body.

Could extra physical activity account for the energy dissipation in the overfeeding experiments? The Ravussin study examined this carefully: the volunteers, when not in the laboratory, wore motion sensors to measure physical activity, and it did not change during overfeeding. And in the study of the young men during *Guru Walla*, they became less active during overfeeding. Anyway, energy use in deliberate physical activity is not exactly what we envisage when we think of someone with fast metabolism, able mysteriously to eat cake and cookies and not gain weight.

Not all physical activity results in obvious external work. James Levine, a professor of medicine at the Mayo Clinic in Rochester, Minnesota, has coined the acronym NEAT for physical activity not associated with 'volitional exercise' such as sports and fitness-related activities. It stands for 'non-exercise activity thermogenesis' – that is, fidgeting, maintenance of posture, and other physical activities of daily life that produce energy in the form of heat. Pointing out that more than three-quarters of the population don't exercise, Levine believes that NEAT is a big factor in the huge variability between people in the total energy they expend, and may explain why some people become obese while others remain lean.[21] With his colleagues, he conducted an overfeeding study in lean volunteers who for eight weeks were given 1,000 kcal per day of food in excess of their normal requirements. All the volunteers gained weight, which was mostly fat with some increase in fat-free mass, but there was large variability in how much individual volunteers gained either fat or fat-free mass: the gain in fat varied from 0.4 kg to 4.2 kg. The experimenters found that the largest component contributing to the differences between the volunteers was NEAT. On average, the increase in NEAT accounted for two-thirds of the increase in daily energy expenditure, but, more importantly, those who increased NEAT the most were those who best resisted weight gain.[22] Levine has gone on to make practical recommendations based on these findings; one is that it is better to stand than to sit while working.[23]

Can we find fast metabolism in the laboratory?

We have looked at various components of metabolism that could explain differences between people in speed of metabolism: differences in energy expenditure in response to eating, or in response to overeating, or natural differences in the ability to burn off fat through brown adipose tissue. We have also seen that non-deliberate physical activity like fidgeting could be why some people can apparently burn off excess energy.

If such differences do exist, we should be able to demonstrate them experimentally, given that they must be rather big differences: comparing someone who can eat unlimited cake and ice cream and not put on weight with someone who struggles to keep the weight off. I am an experimental scientist. I have to ask: can we identify these slow and fast metabolisers, and bring them into the laboratory to find out exactly what makes them tick?

There have been many attempts to do just that. The general idea is to recruit volunteers who claim to be able to eat freely without putting on weight, and to compare them with people who have the opposite view of their metabolic state.

In many earlier studies, people were recruited according to their reported energy intakes, classified as 'low' or 'high' (that is, they were classed as 'small eaters' and 'large eaters'). More recent studies also include reported intakes but recruit people according to how much they feel they have to restrain their eating to avoid putting on weight.

Possibly the first research study to investigate this phenomenon directly was that by Geoffrey Rose and R. Williams
at Paddington General Hospital in London. In 1961 they
published a study using the first approach. The 'large eaters'
reported eating 4,630 kcal/day, whereas the 'small eaters' reported just 2,380 kcal/day; and yet the large eaters weighed
less than the small eaters. Yes, these must surely be 'fast' and
'slow' metabolisers. Rose and Williams measured the energy
expenditure of the subjects at rest, during exercise and after
they had eaten a standard breakfast, but they struggled to find
any real distinction between the two groups. They concluded
that the differences in the energy intakes of the two groups
were 'not due primarily to any constitutional differences in
energy requirements' – in other words, they found no evidence
of fast or slow metabolism.[24]

They were not alone in this finding. More than two decades
later, this issue was addressed more rigorously by Geraldine
McNeill and colleagues at the Rowett Research Institute in
Aberdeen. Musing that 'some individuals are able to eat large
amounts of food without gaining weight, while some others
are less fortunate', they recruited two groups of subjects who
reported widely differing levels of energy intake, and they
measured various components of energy expenditure. But,
once again, they found essentially no differences between the
groups.[25]

Similar findings have come out of many studies. For instance, in two studies published two years apart, a group of
obesity researchers at Laval University in Quebec recruited
'large' and 'small' eaters – in the later study, these were defined
by seven-day diet diaries, with an almost two-fold difference
in reported energy intake. And yet, the investigators noted, the
'large eaters' were lighter than the 'small eaters'. Although the
researchers did consider that there could be a problem with
these reported energy intakes, they concluded that 'it would be

difficult to imagine that errors in reporting could account for the large differences observed in energy intakes between the large eaters and small eaters'.[26] As you may have gathered by now, we can see that they were making the common mistake of placing too much faith in people's ability to record what they were eating.

We see this understanding evolving in a series of papers from researchers at the CSIRO (Australia) Division of Human Nutrition and the Flinders University of South Australia in Adelaide. They described three studies, reported in successive years from 1992. In the first of these, nine 'large-eating' (around 2,900 kcal per day) and nine 'small-eating' (around 1,300 kcal per day) women were selected on the basis of diet and activity diaries. Resting energy expenditure, expressed per kilogram of fat-free mass, was higher by 9–17 per cent in the large eaters compared with the small eaters, although that difference disappeared during exercise.[27] But the following year, the same researchers published a paper titled 'No major differences in energy metabolism between matched and unmatched groups of "large-eating" and "small-eating" men'.[28] Were the findings, just a year later, different because now the subjects were men, not women? Yet the authors also acknowledged a shortcoming in their earlier experiment on women: that the large eaters and small eaters were not matched for body weight. In fact, the large eaters were smaller than the small eaters – as in the studies from Laval University. Just possibly that made the adjustment for fat-free mass unreliable. Finally, in 1994, these researchers published what might be considered the clincher. They measured total energy expenditure using doubly labelled water in groups of 'small eaters' and 'large eaters' (all women again). Now we have experimental measurements outside the confines of the laboratory. The results were clear. The large eaters reported daily energy intakes averaging 2,700 kcal per day, compared with small eaters, who reported 1,340 kcal per day. That's a big difference and should be easily measurable as a difference in energy expenditure. And, indeed, there was a big difference in measured total daily energy expenditure, although it looked rather different: 2,030 kcal per day for the large eaters versus 2,700 kcal per day for the small eaters.[29] (You will see that this is the opposite of what we might expect.) As the experimenters noted, these differences between reported energy intake and measured expenditure should not be sustainable without significant body-weight changes. To hammer home the point, two of the 'small-eating' women were supplied with their reported energy intakes for up to four weeks: both subjects lost about 0.75 kg per week. At the end of this long period of experimentation, the researchers concluded: 'These results provide no support for the existence of "metabolically efficient" women [that is, small eaters, or slow metabolisers] in the community.'

Of several studies comparing those who feel they have to restrain their eating behaviour with those who don't, the largest study that I have come across was published in 2001 by Gaston Bathalon and colleagues at Tufts University, Boston, Massachusetts. They looked at 'non-obese free-living postmenopausal women' classified as long-term restrained eaters (twenty-six women) or unrestrained eaters (thirty-four women). (Oddly, all these studies of 'restraint' involve only women.) They found no difference in energy expenditure between the two groups, either resting energy expenditure or total daily energy expenditure measured with doubly labelled water.[30] Such negative results also came out of other, similar studies.[31]

Still, some studies do find evidence for differences between the restrained and the unrestrained eaters. Reinhard Tuschl and colleagues in Munich began by asking fifty young women to complete a questionnaire which ranked them on the restraint scale. From these women, they selected twelve as restrained eaters and eleven as unrestrained. These women then recorded their normal food intake using diaries, and the restrained eaters did indeed report eating less each day than the unrestrained eaters (2,060 kcal versus 2,300 kcal/day, respectively). Energy expenditure tended to mirror these numbers: per day, restrained 1,960 kcal versus 2,260 kcal/day in the unrestrained.[32] This study did tend to bear out the idea of differences in speed of metabolism (although there has been debate about the validity of the statistics used by the researchers and the physiological plausibility of some of the individual data – some of the unrestrained eaters showed exceptionally high energy expenditures, and some of the restrained, exceptionally low).[33] But another German study with rather similar results perhaps provides an explanation.[34] Rather than claiming that the restrained eaters are such because they have a propensity to put on weight as a result of their perceived slow metabolism, the researchers suggest that their low energy expenditures might be because at least some of them had previously slimmed down from a more over-weight state. We know that a response to a low energy intake is to reduce energy expenditure, as discussed in Chapter 5, and there is some evidence that this effect persists even after weight has stabilised. These women would therefore need restrained eating to maintain their new body weight.

What can we learn from all this? That, when studied in the laboratory, people who claim to be small or restrained eaters, who presumably feel they restrain their eating to keep their body weight in control, may or may not be characterised by a lower energy expenditure than those who don't feel they restrain their eating, the large eaters. And if there is a difference, it is hardly the difference between someone who can eat cream cakes and ice cream and still not gain weight and people who can put on weight on a diet that seems to contain only lettuce leaves. It might even be that the lower energy expenditure, if it exists, is a response to the eating restraint rather than vice versa.

Fast and slow metabolism – an elusive phenomenon

We have been looking specifically at whether there are some people with an intrinsically fast metabolism, and some who are metabolically challenged the opposite way – a common perception. We have seen that, although metabolic mechanisms exist that could explain this variation, they do not seem to operate in humans as they do in rodents. These differences in metabolic speed are remarkably hard to pin down when people are brought into the laboratory.

What these observations do tell us, once again, is that it is very easy to get a false impression of how much, or how little, any one person is eating – and scientists don't do much better when they supposedly capture this behaviour by recording it. But, as we have seen, acceptance of this fact has been slow – hence prestigious institutions still insisting that there are those who can have their cake and eat it. None of this is to say that there are not differences in metabolic speed. Like all human qualities, there will be variation among people in energy expenditure, just as there are differences in height, blood pressure or ability to do press-ups. Indeed, researchers often make a point of stressing the amount of variability in energy expenditure between people. But it just doesn't seem to relate to people's reported food intake, or their need to restrain their eating. The ability to eat cream cakes and not gain weight, although a vivid impression in our minds, turns out to be a remarkably elusive phenomenon.

Of course, there are the extreme few who still struggle to

eat enough to maintain their weight. They are mostly elite sportspeople, mountaineers and polar explorers. They – and the majority of us who at most might exercise with a slow jog around the park – will be our focus in Chapter 8, after we've looked at how misled we were for many years over the causes of obesity.

7

The riddle of obesity

Obesity has been with us for a long time. A series of small carved figures from Palaeolithic times and later has been discovered in various sites across Europe, depicting mainly obese females, and known as Venuses. In 2009 Nicholas Conard, an American-German archaeologist, reported in the journal *Nature* the discovery of one such figurine in south-western Germany. This figurine dates from 35,000 years ago, 'making it one of the oldest known examples of figurative art'.[1] It was for a long time thought that these early figurines were representations of pregnant women, and hence perhaps fertility symbols, but this view has changed, and many now consider that these are, indeed, representations of obesity.[2]

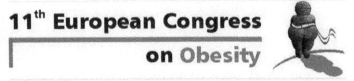

The 30,000-year-old Venus of Willendorf, adopted as the mascot of the 11th European Congress on Obesity, Vienna, 2001.

Several millennia later, in his 'Discourse concerning the causes and effects of corpulence' published in 1728, the English physician Thomas Short wrote, 'I believe no age did ever afford more instances of corpulency than our own.'[3] But today, in westernised societies, there is no doubt that obesity is increasing at an unprecedented and alarming rate. According to the World Health Organization (WHO), 'Worldwide obesity has nearly tripled since 1975. In 2016, more than 1.9 billion adults ... were overweight. Of these over 650 million were obese. Most of the world's population live in countries where overweight and obesity kills more people than underweight.'[4]

Nevertheless, we argue about the causes of obesity. Despite the arguments I put forward in the previous chapter, many people still wish to believe in their 'slow metabolism'. Experts argue that we have not been able to stop the increase in obesity because we've been working on false assumptions: that it's not as simple as 'calories in–calories out'. But the problem is, as I have now been arguing over several chapters, that we have grave difficulties in assessing how much we, as individuals, or others, eat – leading to confusion that has dogged the field of obesity research for a long time.

Body fat – and other measures

The WHO defines obesity as abnormal or excessive fat accumulation that may impair health. Excessive fat accumulation markedly increases the risk of many conditions, including type-2 diabetes, coronary heart disease and certain cancers – and, in general, the more the fat accumulation, the greater the risk.

If I were a doctor, how would I know if my patient was

obese? How much fat would count as abnormal or excessive? And how do we measure fat content in the first place?

For just £25, I can buy a 'diagnostic' bathroom scale that will tell me both my weight and the amount of fat in my body. But until two decades or so ago, specialised facilities were required to measure body fat. One traditional technique is underwater weighing – essentially involving a large water tank and a weighing scale.* Because fat is less dense than other tissues, if we can measure the density of the whole body, we can work out the content of fat and other components. There are also simpler, if less specific, methods. In 1974, John Durnin and John Womersley in Glasgow published measurements of body fat by underwater weighing in nearly 500 adults and compared these results with measurements of skinfold thickness using a calliper to pinch the skin. They did this at four sites on the body: two on the upper arm, one below the shoulder blade and one just above the hip. Because the thickness of the pinch is a good indicator of the amount of fat under the skin, they could use skinfold measurements to estimate body fat in men and women of different ages.[5] Today, there are various methods, including measuring the body's electrical resistance (since fat does not conduct electricity) – which is how those bathroom scales work – and an X-ray technique that distinguishes fat from other tissues (called dual-energy X-ray absorptiometry, or DXA), now a gold standard for fat measurement.

In most large studies of obesity, however, the measure used is body mass index, or BMI: the body weight in kilograms divided by the square of the height in metres. This measure was first introduced by a Belgian astronomer and

---

* The apparent loss in weight when a body is weighed in air and in water is equal to the weight of water displaced – Archimedes' principle. The weight of water displaced gives the volume of the body, and the weight in air then gives the density. A correction is made for air in the lungs.

statistician, Adolphe Quetelet, in 1869. He collated data on the Belgian population, especially studying changes in height and weight as people grow. He tried correcting weight by dividing by height, then discovered that if he corrected by dividing by the square of height, he obtained similar values for people of similar build, whatever their height. ('Similar build' implies a similar percentage body fat, which is what we want to compare.) This measure was called Quetelet's index until the American nutritionist Ancel Keys named it body mass index in 1972. The WHO classifies those with a BMI over 25 kg/m² as overweight, and those with a BMI greater than 30 kg/m² as obese. Before dealing with other criticisms of BMI as a measure of fatness, we should note that the measure was based on the then-white population of Belgium, and these cut-offs may not be appropriate for people of other ethnicities.

Some argue that BMI is misleading because it doesn't directly measure body fat – just body weight. A muscular individual – a sportsperson, for example – might have a small amount of body fat but a high BMI because of the weight of their muscles. This must be true. But is it a big confounding factor? We can look at some published data for elite sportspeople. The average BMI of the eight-man Oxford crew for the 2022 annual rowing race between Cambridge and Oxford universities was 24.7 kg/m² – not even what we would categorise as overweight. And these are big, muscular guys you would not want to mess with. When the British boxer Tyson Fury retained his World Heavyweight Championship in 2022, the media reported on his statistics, along with those of Rocky Marciano, whom many regard as the best heavyweight boxer of all time. Their respective BMIs were 28.9 and 25.5 kg/m². Yes, I agree, almost certainly these chaps had low body fat and were jumped into the 'overweight' category by their muscle bulk.

We see this taken to extremes in some cases. The American footballer Daniel Faalele 'is set to become the heaviest player in the NFL [National Football League] after being drafted by Baltimore Ravens', according to BBC News, and he has a BMI of 42.2 kg/m². And the top five contenders in the World's Strongest Man competition of 2021 have an average BMI of 43 kg/m². I'm sure none of these individuals carries excess fat. But they are real bodybuilders.

Although a lot of muscle can clearly distort the BMI, this is not the case for the general population, where there is a strikingly close relationship between body fat and both body weight and BMI (see illustration opposite). It's important to note that we may accumulate many, many kilograms of fat. From the graph we can see that a man with a BMI of 40 kg/m² will have (on average) 49 kg of fat, whereas a man with a BMI of 20 kg/m² will have (again on average) just 10 kg of fat – almost a five-fold difference. (The pattern is similar for women, although not so pronounced.) Having said that, it's true that we cannot predict how much fat someone carries precisely from their BMI. For a BMI of 25 kg/m², women on the graph have between 16 and 30 kg of fat. But those are the extremes: most lie closer to the middle of the distribution shown on the graph. If you are someone who regularly lifts weights in the gym, yes, your BMI will be higher because of your muscle bulk, and your build would be more accurately assessed by measuring body composition. But for most people in the general population, 'It's all down to my big muscles' probably ranks alongside 'big bones' as an explanation for excess weight.

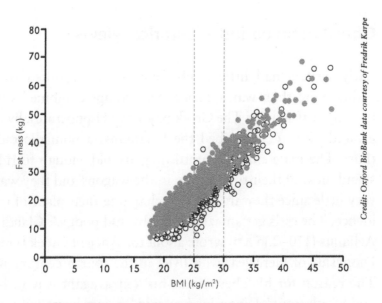

A graph of body fat (in kg) plotted against BMI for 1,500 people randomly selected from the Oxfordshire population. The dashed vertical lines show conventional cut-offs for defining overweight (BMI above 25 kg/m^2) and obesity (BMI above 30 kg/m^2). Filled dots represent women; open dots, men.

There is now a strong body of opinion that BMI does not necessarily equate directly to the risk of metabolic diseases; this may be better captured by measures such as waist circumference – assessing more specifically fat in the abdominal area. Fat in the lower part of the body – thighs and legs – doesn't have the same relationship to metabolic changes such as the risk of type-2 diabetes. It's something we have worked on in our laboratory.[6] The reason is partly to do with the different nature of the fat (more 'inflammatory changes' occur in abdominal fat), and also the fact that fat in the abdominal area is not just under the skin, it's within the abdomen around internal organs, where it may have adverse effects. But in this chapter we will stick to overall body fat, usually as assessed by BMI, as this is most relevant to our calorie balance and weight.

Obesity and eating – historical views

Early writers had little doubt that obesity resulted from eating more than was appropriate, perhaps combined with less physical activity. The Greek physician Hippocrates, living around 400 BC, described the Scythians, a nomadic race, thus: 'The male children, until they are old enough to ride, spend most of their time sitting in the wagons and they walk very little since they are so often changing their place of residence. The girls get amazingly flabby and podgy.'[7] Claudius Aelianus (170–235 AD) wrote about the Ancient Greek tyrant Dionysius of Heraclea, who lived in the fourth century BC. The reason for his obesity was his 'extravagant way of life and his gluttony'. Dionysius was said 'to be ashamed of himself and lived secluded in a small tower where he developed a huge body'.[8] Ibn Sina, known in the West as Avicenna (980–1037 AD), recognised the predisposition of 'hugely obese persons' to fall ill quickly and recommended heavy exercise on an empty stomach.[9] Samuel Pepys, in seventeenth-century London, describes many 'fat' people, such as Mrs Lane, to whom he had evidently taken a fancy, and whom he did 'so touse her and feel her all over, making her believe how fair and good a skin she has, and indeed she has a very white thigh and leg, but monstrous fat'. But he does not generally discuss why these people have become 'fat', although when he meets his old school friend, Mr Christmas, he notes: 'but a deadly drinker he is, and grown exceeding fat'.[10] (Pepys reminds us that calories from alcohol all count towards our calorie balance.)

All this fits with the explanation for obesity provided by the energy balance model: obesity arises when, over a prolonged period, energy intake exceeds energy expenditure and the body's fat stores increase to the point where there are health risks. But why does intake exceed expenditure? Is it because intake is unduly high, or because energy expenditure is low?

As we will see in the rest of this chapter, our understanding of obesity has changed dramatically over the past five decades. We now have a clearer view of what is happening to the energetics of the body when it is on a trajectory of gaining weight, or even when at a steady, but overgenerous, weight – explaining why it's so difficult to shed the excess pounds. But first we need to look at early studies that cast doubt on the calorie-balance model by suggesting that obesity was not due to overeating – and confront a recurring theme in this book: that attempts to record what people eat may be seriously misleading.

Overeating, underreporting

In 1972, Jetson E. Lincoln (vice president of finance and planning at the international tobacco company, Philip Morris USA) reviewed several studies of the relationship between energy intake and obesity, and concluded that 'the popular idea that obesity is usually the result of overeating is not supported in the literature'. One of the studies he examined was that by Rose and Williams in London, that we looked at in the last chapter. As we saw, they recruited pairs of participants who, according to dietary questionnaires, ate very different amounts: but the 'small eaters' were heavier than the 'large eaters'. Lincoln went on to conduct his own 'questionnaire study of food and beverage intake among 867 men', which, he claimed, indicated that the more obese consumed no more calories than the less obese groups. 'This appeared to be due to restraint on their part rather than lack of appetite', he argued.[11]

Around the same time, biological mechanisms were being

described that could contribute to low energy expenditure – in other words, slow metabolism. Jean Himms-Hagen at the University of Ottawa wrote: 'For obesity to occur, energy intake must exceed energy expenditure. Yet some people may indulge in gluttony and sloth with impunity, others only with unwelcome consequences; still others may not indulge at all but nevertheless become obese' – and went on to suggest that obesity may be caused by a defect in the brown fat's ability to burn off energy.[12] George Blackburn, Jeffrey Flier and Mario de Luise at Harvard Medical School described obesity as 'a clinical situation in which disordered cellular thermogenesis [that is, the ability of cells to burn off energy as heat] may have a critical role' and demonstrated a defect associated with obesity in the pump that moves sodium and potassium ions across cell membranes. This pump, crucial for nerve signals, heart beats and muscle contractions, among other things, is a major user of energy in cells.[13]

I came across these ideas through Harry Keen, a world expert in diabetes at Guy's Hospital Medical School, London, whom I first met when he was my PhD thesis examiner in the 1970s. At Guy's, Harry worked closely with the epidemiologist John Jarrett on the risk factors for heart disease and diabetes. In 1979 they published a paper entitled 'Nutrient intake, adiposity, and diabetes'. They analysed data from three large studies of 'normal populations', nearly 3,000 people in all. In each of these studies, the participants had made a record of dietary intake over a period of one to three days. The authors looked at the relationship between dietary energy intake and BMI. They found that the bigger people were, the less they seemed to eat, and concluded that a key mechanism leading to human obesity was 'slow metabolism'.[14]

Several other studies around this time pointed to the same conclusion. In 1978, Daan Kromhout, a Dutch expert on the epidemiology of cardiovascular disease, became the lead investigator in a long-term study of a cohort of several hundred men that began in the 1960s and continues to this day: the Zutphen Study. In a 1983 paper, he started by stating that obese individuals in affluent cultures generally have a lower energy intake than their lean counterparts. He then looked at data from 800 men in the cohort to confirm this view, and particularly to discover which nutrients the overweight men were under-consuming. He found that the most obese men reported eating 300 kcal a day less than the leanest men. The energy intake per kilogram of body weight was 35.7 kcal/kg in the obese, against 51.4 kcal/kg in the lean. This difference was reflected in each of the macronutrients – carbohydrates, fat and protein – but he noted that the obese men drank more alcohol than the lean.[15] A year later, researchers from Laval University in Quebec conducted a similar study that looked at both children and adults in families. They also found that greater weight was associated with lower reported intake of energy. As in Kromhout's study, this reduction was spread evenly over the major nutrients (and, curiously, alcohol intake was again positively related to fatness). The researchers concluded that their results also supported the idea that heavier individuals generally consume fewer calories than their lean counterparts.[16]

We now know that these studies were invariably flawed by the difficulty of obtaining reliable measurements of what people are eating – and the failure of the scientists of the time to recognise this difficulty. This is the issue of underreporting that we examined in Chapter 3. We are now aware of potential pitfalls and biases that researchers then simply didn't appreciate. With hindsight, we can understand why in 1976 highly respected contemporaries of mine, Phil James and Paul Trayhurn, both obesity experts, wrote in the *Lancet*: 'A few obese individuals ingesting huge amounts of energy are known to every physician. Nevertheless, the formal studies of food intake usually show that most obese subjects do not eat more than their slim counterparts.'[17]

The difficulty of knowing what people are eating was exemplified in a 1986 study by Andrew Prentice and colleagues at the Dunn Clinical Nutrition Centre in Cambridge – at the time world experts in measuring food intake. The researchers, who were looking at energy expenditure in lean and obese women, noted: 'Each subject recorded her food intake by weighing all foods and fluids over seven days for the lean group and over two periods of seven days for the obese group.' That sounds intensive. Yet the results speak for themselves. The reported energy intake for the group of lean women was, on average, 98 per cent of their measured energy expenditure – a testament to the care taken over the experiments. But, for the group of obese women, reported energy intake was 66 per cent of measured expenditure; in fact, it was considerably lower than the reported intake for the lean women. If this reported intake were true, then the women would have been losing weight fast – which they weren't.[18]

What lies behind underreporting of energy intake? In the early 2000s, my research group in Oxford was part of a consortium with obesity researchers in Cambridge. Our aim was to study the 'integrative physiology' of obesity and diabetes – looking at the broader interactions of body systems as well as the cellular and molecular details. One of the requirements of our funder, the Wellcome Trust, was that we include a training programme for younger researchers. At our annual consortium meetings, we would plan a session for the junior scientists, including a presentation of various dilemmas which the juniors would then discuss among themselves, before presenting their thinking to the wider audience. One problem we set was that of a patient who complains to their doctor about steady weight gain despite eating very little. We asked, 'What investigations would you do?' The first young researcher started by saying, 'Well, he's lying.' He was immediately slammed down. In one sense his claim must be true, but it's probably not a case of deliberately concealing information – as I described in Chapter 3, even I, with an interest in getting the right answers, have found that I may record something that's not typical of my daily diet. Rather, I suspect the reason overweight people tend to under-report more than lean people may be intrinsic to their biological make-up. As we saw in Chapter 5, and will examine further below, there's a strong inherited tendency to obesity or leanness, and the genes involved act almost exclusively on pathways regulating appetite rather than speed of metabolism. Perhaps part of this genetic influence involves altering our ability to recognise just what we are eating.

Asking what people are eating is clearly not going to help us understand the causes of obesity. Fortunately, there's another way of finding this out. For someone whose weight is not changing drastically from day to day, their energy intake must, on average, match their energy expenditure – that's the energy balance model. If obesity is due to a metabolic defect – slow metabolism – then we'd expect that person's energy expenditure to be low. As we've seen, for several decades now we've been able to measure energy expenditure very accurately over long periods in people leading their daily lives – and these studies have revealed something that at first glance is rather surprising about energy expenditure and obesity.

Faster metabolisers

In the early 1980s a young Swiss obesity researcher, Eric Ravussin, with colleagues at the Institute of Physiology at the University of Lausanne, looked at energy expenditure in three groups of people: 'obese' and 'moderately obese' individuals as well as lean controls. (Ravussin later made a career in the USA: we have looked at his work a few times and will do so again.) The volunteers were studied in a calorimetry chamber, and their total energy expenditure measured over twenty-four hours. The researchers also measured energy expenditure while the volunteers were resting quietly after an overnight fast. The results are shown in the table below (figures reproduced with permission).

	Mean BMI kg/m²	Resting energy expenditure	24-hour energy expenditure
Lean	21	1,460	2,020
Moderately obese	26	1,590	2,290
Obese	38	1,810	2,400

Energy expenditure in people in the calorimetry chamber. Measurements of energy expenditure are in kcal per twenty-four hours. (I have calculated the BMI from mean height and weight.)[19]

There was a clear pattern: the larger the person, the greater their energy expenditure, not just during daytime, when the extra energy cost of moving a heavier body might have been relevant, but also at rest and during sleep. This went against the popular belief in slow metabolism. In fact, the results showed *fast* metabolism in obese people. What could that mean?

The energy balance model tells us that an increased energy expenditure must be matched by an increased energy intake – provided that the person is in a roughly steady metabolic state. Which means that, for most obese people, the driver for maintaining their obesity is not *limited* energy expenditure, but *increased* energy intake.

Why, then, is energy expenditure greater in obese people than lean? The answer, suggested by Ravussin and colleagues, is that as well as increased fat mass, obese people have increased lean mass compared with lean people. Again, this won't apply to everyone: there are muscular lean people, as we've seen. But it is true on average.

When we measure body fat content, we are not talking about the amount of adipose tissue; rather, we are talking about the amount of chemical fat throughout the body. By far the majority of this is in the fat cells in adipose tissue, although there is also some in many other tissues, such as the fat that acts as nerve insulation in the brain. Stored fat is metabolically inert: it is just there as a reserve in case of starvation (or has other functions, as in the brain) and does not contribute to resting metabolic rate. The remainder of our body weight is our non-fat mass, often called fat-free mass or lean body mass. That includes the bones, which are also relatively metabolically inert.*

Lean body mass refers to all tissues and parts of cells that are not fat – essentially the water-containing part of the body. In fact, one way to measure it is to give the volunteer a dose of water labelled with an isotope (for example, water made up of oxygen and deuterium, a heavier form of hydrogen – sometimes called 'heavy water'), and measure how much it is diluted in the body. It includes the major organs – liver, intestines, kidneys, muscles, heart, and so on – but also the water component of the fatty tissues, including brain and adipose tissue. These are the parts of

---

* In some measures of lean body mass, bone mass is also subtracted from total body weight, but usually this is not the case. Today, as dual-energy X-ray absorptiometry, DXA, is used to assess body composition, this becomes easier. DXA was originally introduced to measure bone density – if you ever need to have a bone scan to check for osteoporosis, this will be done with a DXA machine. Nowadays it is therefore easier to assess the true non-fat, non-bone mass – but in the studies I am looking at here, this was not usually done.

the body in which metabolism is using fuel, and energy is being liberated.

Ravussin and colleagues found that their obese volunteers had greater fat-free mass than the lean – 63 kg in the obese group compared with 49 kg in the lean. This makes sense: adipose tissue itself contains material other than fat (around 10–15 per cent of its weight is not fat), and connective tissues must also increase to support the additional fat mass. They noted that energy expenditure varied with fat-free mass: if they divided 24-hour energy expenditure by fat-free mass, the results were similar in lean and obese people. In other words, obese people had a higher energy expenditure than lean because of their higher fat-free mass.

These studies were made under strictly controlled conditions. The participants were confined to the laboratory and the investigations were only for short periods. If we want to understand how much energy people expend during their usual daily lives, we need an alternative method. We could ask them to wear portable sampling devices, as was done in the early studies on army recruits that we looked at in Chapter 3. But that might affect what they do. This is where the doubly labelled water method (described in Chapter 2) comes in. It enables the investigator to measure total energy expenditure over a period of two to three weeks while the volunteer is living a normal life: just perhaps popping into the laboratory every few days to provide a sample, although even that is not necessary – the volunteer can just collect small samples of saliva or urine in pots for later analysis.

In their 1986 study, Prentice and colleagues used this method to measure energy expenditure in the lean and obese women living their normal daily lives. Their results were like those obtained by Ravussin. They found a strong relationship between fat-free mass and energy expenditure (both resting in the calorimeter chamber, and free living, measured over two to four weeks): in other words, fat-free mass appeared to govern energy expenditure. And more to the point, they found that free-living energy expenditure was considerably higher in the obese than in the lean women: the obese women expended an average of 28 per cent more energy than the lean controls. The only possible conclusion is that the obese women were also eating considerably more than the lean.

All these studies were of people who were already obese. They do not show how obesity begins to develop. Conceivably, there is an initial defect in metabolism that leads to expansion of the fat stores, somehow in turn then resetting energy expenditure to higher levels. In fact, this is what James and Trayhurn proposed in their 1976 *Lancet* article. But – in acknowledging that some studies were showing high rates of energy expenditure in obese people – they suggested that 'the enlargement of the adipocytes during the development of obesity leads to an increase in the energy expended, and the BMR [basal metabolic rate, or resting energy expenditure] rises'. In other words, they were proposing an initial defect that we might characterise as slow metabolism, changing to a picture of elevated energy expenditure as the fat cells expand.

John Garrow, with Joan Webster, addressed this idea in a study published in 1985, titled 'Are pre-obese people energy thrifty?' They studied energy expenditure in women with a wide range of body fat. They argued that if energy expenditure were measured and expressed in relation to the fat-free mass, this should unmask the intrinsic metabolic defect that James and Trayhurn had proposed. But they could find no evidence for such a defect, leading them to conclude (using the language of their time): 'It is difficult to believe that fat people with a high metabolic rate relative to fat-free mass once had a low metabolic rate.'[20]

In the end, though, we need studies that follow people over

many years as obesity develops. In a long-term study from the National Institute on Aging in Baltimore, USA, published in 1995, the researchers made detailed measurements of 775 men, then followed them for ten years to track their weight. They found a weak relationship between initial resting energy expenditure and subsequent weight gain – but not in the expected direction. Those with lower resting energy expenditure tended to gain the least weight. There was no evidence that some people showed slow metabolism and then tended to gain more weight.[21] A similar result was found in the Quebec family study from Laval University, albeit with a shorter, five-and-a-half-year follow-up; the investigators reviewed other similar studies and generally found no such relationship.[22]

Mind the gap

During a long career teaching metabolism to medical students, I gradually introduced more on the topic of obesity as it became a bigger public-health issue. I used to set the students a little calculation to look at how obesity might develop. (It's closely related to the calculation I presented on page 85 in Chapter 5 about the precision of energy balance.) It typically took them several minutes, allowing me to collect my thoughts, before some, often bizarre, answers emerged. The task went as follows.

A twenty-year-old student, weighing 65 kg, has a daily energy intake and daily energy expenditure of 2,400 kcal. They therefore remain at a constant body weight. After graduating, they take a job in the city, and commute to work by car instead of cycling or walking. This reduces energy expenditure by 190 kcal per day, for five days per week. If their energy intake does not also change, what will their weight be at the age of forty? (I used to point out also that the last assumption was probably unrealistic: city lunches, after-work drinks, dinner gatherings, and so on, are likely to increase energy consumption compared with impoverished student life.)

A rough calculation is as follows. The energy gain each week (five days) is 190 × 5 kcal, or 950 kcal/week; with (say) fifty working weeks per year that's 950 × 50 kcal or 47,500 kcal per year; over twenty years, 47,500 × 20 kcal or 950,000 kcal is gained. Each kilogram of adipose tissue stores about 7,000 kcal of energy, so 950,000 kcal equates to 950,000 ÷7,000 kg, or around 135 kg of weight gain: the student turned business executive has gained about 200 per cent in body weight over twenty years – and now weighs three times as much as when a student.

'Oh, but that's unrealistic,' the students would say: yet, when challenged to say exactly which bit is unrealistic, they, and I, failed.

This calculation is similar to an illustration given by Reg Passmore in 1971:

> Imagine a healthy man or woman, who either eats an extra half slice of bread (50 g) at breakfast or takes his car to work instead of walking (10 min each way) and goes into a positive energy balance of 50 kcal/day. If there are no compensatory changes he or she will store in 10 years an extra 20 kg of tri-glyceride [triacylglycerol, in fat cells] and be seriously obese. It is not necessary to be a glutton to become obese.[23]

A similar illustration attributed to Passmore starts, 'Imagine there are two twins; one begins to add an extra pat of butter each day to their breakfast toast' – and then goes on to calculate, in a similar way, the huge cumulative energy gain.*

---

* This was told to me by Romaine Hervey, whose work on rats we met in Chapter 5. I cannot now trace its source.

Like my teaching example, though, Passmore's calculations were wrong. Data from the study of obese and lean people in Lausanne (see the table 'Energy expenditure in people in the calorimetry chamber' on page 140) show that the difference in 24-hour energy expenditure between them is about 380 kcal per day. In the study by Prentice and colleagues it was about 525 kcal per day. These figures are much more than Passmore's suggested 'extra pat of butter each day', or my calculation of a difference of about 190 kcal per day leading to a tripling of weight.

The problem with the simplistic calculations done by Passmore and my students is that they ignore the fact that, as weight increases, part of that weight is fat-free mass, so energy expenditure will also increase. This may be a natural result of growing the body's mass, but it is hard not to see it as a mechanism that has evolved to stabilise body weight, just as the fall in energy expenditure with reduction of energy intake tends to stabilise weight the other way.

This was clarified for me some years ago by the work of Kevin Hall at the National Institute of Diabetes and Digestive and Kidney Diseases in Bethesda, Maryland, USA. Kevin has studied the metabolism of obese people. He started in research as a mathematician, taking data from published studies, including some of my work on adipose tissue metabolism, and creating mathematical models that explain them. More recently, he has also led experimental approaches to weight loss. In 2010 the editors of the *Lancet* commissioned a series of review papers relating to obesity. Hall and his colleagues were asked to write a paper on energy balance. Eric Ravussin and I were asked to be expert reviewers at a meeting in London – to challenge the authors and help them improve their papers. We had some comments to make on Hall's paper, largely about the difficulty for non-mathematically minded readers of understanding some of the models used. But the substance of the paper remained unchanged, and provided important insights even for supposed experts such as myself, who had struggled to understand exactly what goes on as obesity develops.

The main thrust of the paper was to show the dynamics of weight change in response to a change in energy balance, whether brought about by a change in energy intake or in physical activity. Hall pointed out that changes in body weight in response to a change in energy balance are slower than most of us would expect. But the results I want to highlight were an attempt by the authors to model what happened to the US population during the rapid development of the obesity epidemic. They took data from the National Health and Nutrition Examination Survey (NHANES) of the US population from 1978 to 2005. These show a steady increase in the average body weight of the US population, from around 71 kg to 81 kg. They used their models to calculate that this increase in body weight would result from a daily excess of energy intake over expenditure of just 7 kcal per day – that really is Passmore's 'extra pat of butter'. This is what Hall refers to as the 'energy imbalance gap'. But, as weight increased, so did energy expenditure: from around 2,390 kcal per day to 2,630 kcal – an increase of 240 kcal per day. This is referred to as the 'maintenance energy gap'. Energy intake must have increased by 240 kcal/day over the same period, but all the time remained just 7 kcal per day above energy expenditure. This increase in energy intake of about 240 kcal per day over the 27 years is an average figure across the adult US population – not individual data. The increase in energy intake will have been much greater in those gaining more weight than average, so these figures tie in with observations from Ravussin and Prentice and others.[24] How should we interpret this? Someone might begin with a small daily surplus of energy – literally that extra pat of butter, or a little less exercise. That's enough to start the increase in body weight. But as the body weight increases, so does the fat-free mass; and, along with this, energy expenditure rises. This could be seen as a natural compensatory mechanism. A person will only keep gaining weight, though, if their energy intake gradually increases so that it remains greater than energy expenditure. After say twenty to thirty years, the increase in intake from the starting point is significant (perhaps as much as 500 kcal per day). If that person wants to return to their original weight, that's the magnitude of the challenge: not to drop daily energy intake by 7 kcal, or a pat of butter per day, but by 500 kcal – about a Big Mac's worth.

Genes and the rapid increase in obesity

We saw in Chapter 5 that there is a strong genetic tendency towards obesity. The offspring of obese parents are likely themselves to accumulate excess weight, and this goes beyond the shared family traits of preparing food and eating.

Nevertheless, our genetic background has not changed in the past thirty years or so. How, then, can genetics explain the sudden increase in obesity over this period? The answer is that genes exert their effects according to the environment. If food is scarce, there will still be genetically induced variation in body weight in the population, but the whole distribution will be skewed towards leanness rather than obesity. When food is plentiful, and a sedentary lifestyle predominates, the distribution will shift towards the heavier end: still, genetics will govern (to a greater or lesser extent) where an individual lies within that distribution. It seems to me that this is exactly what I have seen happening over my lifetime.

As we saw in Chapter 5, there are some individual genes that have been proven to play a role in obesity or leanness, together with a large number of genetic variations that play very minor roles. But it remains true that, in so far as we understand the functions of the genes involved, they are in the pathways of appetite regulation – energy intake – rather than energy expenditure. That really does not in any way change our understanding of the causes of obesity.

Energy balance and obesity in perspective

Our understanding of obesity has changed dramatically over the past five decades. We now accept that over-consumption of energy underlies almost all human obesity: and that a large component of over-consumption is genetically determined. But although the basis of obesity as a disorder of energy balance cannot be disputed, there are still plenty of challenges to the idea that this is as simple as some people eating more than others. And, of course, there is some truth in that. Although I hope I have dismissed the idea of lucky people who can burn off cakes and ice cream without having to think about it, we can all increase our energy expenditure in a very conscious way: through physical activity. But just how much can physical activity change our energy use? That demands a quantitative look at energy expenditure during activity.

8

Let's get moving! Physical activity and calorie balance

It was summer in 1992 when the British explorer Sir Ranulph Fiennes and his companion Dr Mike Stroud stepped out of the Twin Otter plane onto the Filchner ice shelf on the Atlantic coast of Antarctica. Ninety-six days later, they were flown out from the Ross ice shelf, having crossed the continent, covering 2,300 km without any external support, pulling all their equipment and supplies on sledges.

Mike Stroud is a physician, scientist and inveterate explorer. He had been on two previous expeditions with Fiennes, attempting to reach the North Pole unsupported – that is, with no external assistance once they had left their base camp. Each time they had had to give up – on the second occasion, just a couple of degrees of latitude short of the Pole, because they were running out of food, Stroud was beginning to hallucinate, as his blood sugar dropped, and Fiennes was having quite different problems with his eyes.[1]

The experience from these expeditions had shown Mike Stroud what they needed to do in the Antarctic. There was a compromise to be made. They knew that their energy expenditure would be very high, dragging sledges over the ice and up to the high Antarctic plateau. But the more food they carried, the heavier the sledges became, The answer? Stroud devised rations that were high in calories and as low in weight as possible. In practice, that meant that they had to be fat-rich, with butter and chocolate providing much of the energy. It is a principle that we will look at again later (in Chapter 11), that fat adds to the energy density of food (kcal per kilogram). This was helpful for the explorers but may not be so good for those of us not pulling sledges in the wilderness.

Stroud made scientific measurements during the expedition. He knew exactly what they were each eating, and so calculated energy intake. They took in, on average, just over 5,000 kcal/day. He also measured energy expenditure with doubly labelled water, described in Chapter 2. Over the whole expedition, energy expenditure averaged 6,000–7,000 kcal/day. During the hardest phase, dragging the sledges uphill from the ice shelf to the high plateau, energy expenditure was remarkably high: 11,000–12,000 kcal/day. Clearly, the two men were in considerable negative energy balance – as they had expected to be – and lost large amounts of weight (14 and 10 kg respectively), and their body-fat stores, measured when they returned, had dropped to extremely low levels – almost unmeasurable.

This expedition provided a very clear example of just what our fat stores are for: without reasonable fat stores to begin with, these men could never have completed the trek. It also shows just how physical exercise increases our energy expenditure.[2]

Another extreme study was conducted by Klaas Westerterp of the University of Maastricht. Klaas is himself a fit mountain walker, but in the laboratory he is one of the world experts in measuring energy expenditure using the doubly labelled water technique. He studied a group of five people who were planning to climb Mount Everest. He made measurements during their training in the Alps, then during the ascent at high altitude – including 'observations ... on Mount Everest just before the summit was reached in three subjects, and including the summit (8,872 metres) in a fourth'. The introduction to the paper Westerterp and colleagues published on this study points out, with understatement, 'it is difficult to perform energy balance studies under field conditions at sea level [as we have seen with Edholm's studies of cadets in Chapter 3]. Living in camps at high altitude further complicates the measurements.' Energy expenditure was measured with the doubly labelled water technique, so the results are an average over the experimental period – we don't know how high the energy expenditure was when actually climbing. Averages over twenty-four hours were: energy intake, 1,800 kcal/day, energy expenditure, 3,250 kcal/day. This seems a low energy intake for strenuous exercise, and indeed during the training phase in the Alps average intake was greater at 2,410 kcal/day, whereas energy expenditure was 3,510 kcal/day. Energy intake was probably low because of the extreme conditions. Clearly, energy expenditure was much higher than intake, similar to other studies in strenuous exercise, and all the climbers lost weight – as we would expect.[3] Jonas Enqvist in Sweden measured energy intake and expenditure in nine men taking part in an 800 km 'adventure race' involving running, mountain biking, kayaking, inline skating, climbing, caving and canyoneering, with a total exercise time of just over six days. Energy expenditure over that period was 80,000 kcal (12,000 kcal/day on average). Intake was difficult to measure, but it was clear that the athletes were struggling to take in sufficient calories, and this was reflected in a 2 kg fall in body-fat content.[4]

My own small contribution to this field of energy balance during exertion came about when, in the late 1990s, with colleagues in Liverpool and Manchester, I was awarded a research grant from the Mars Corporation to look at 'Nutritional and energetic aspects of hill walking'. (My colleagues, knowing of my personal interest in mountain walking, thought this a great joke.) We appointed a PhD student, Phil Ainslie, to conduct the studies. Phil had qualifications in both human physiology and mountain leadership. (He is now a Professor at the University of British Columbia.) For his first experiments, he persuaded volunteers, on separate days, to walk with him up Bowfell, a 902-metre-high hill in the English Lake District. While they walked, often in atrocious weather, the volunteers breathed into a mask to measure oxygen consumption (and hence energy expenditure) via a portable apparatus in a backpack (the Metamax system shown on page 48, 'Measuring energy expenditure during activity with a backpack apparatus'). Since Phil controlled the energy supply (he provided the food for the volunteers), he knew their energy intake. A summary was that energy intake – breakfast and lunch – averaged 1,300 kcal, whereas energy expenditure was 3,470 kcal.[5] The volunteers were in very clear negative energy balance during the walk. (Of course, they may well have made it up with a good evening meal, and perhaps a pint of beer.) Phil then persuaded two groups of men, 'younger' (average age of twenty-four years) and 'older' (fifty-six years), to join him on a trip to the Scottish Highlands, where he measured energy expenditure during ten days of strenuous hill walking, averaging 21 kilometres in distance and 1,160 metres of ascent each day. Not only did Klaas Westerterp, mentioned above, make the measurements of energy expenditure in this study using doubly labelled water but he was also one of the participants. To our surprise, average energy expenditure was 5,000–5,300 kcal/day, much higher than we had expected, and comparable with figures for ultra-marathon runners in a twenty-day, 500 km road race, and lumberjacks in Maine, USA. The men managed heroic energy intakes of 3,600–4,500 kcal/day, but still all lost weight and body fat.[6]

Elite athletes are well aware of their energy requirements, and modern sports science places great weight on meeting those energy needs. Scientists at the University of Maastricht (Klaas Westerterp's own institution) have looked at elite cyclists taking part in the Tour de France, a three-week event in which the competitors then covered 4,000 km including thirty mountain stages, with only one rest day and one shorter time-trial day. Initially, they invited cyclists into the laboratory. In Maastricht they have two indirect calorimetry chambers, each large enough for an elite cyclist to live inside for seven days, along with a stationary bicycle. The experimenters set up a simulation of the Tour de France. This experience was used to look at energy expenditure in the various stages, as well as nutritional needs. Then the Maastricht group followed four riders in detail during the actual event. Energy expenditure was extraordinarily high during the days spent climbing in the mountains: up to 7,900 kcal. But then there was a rest day and a shorter day, when energy expenditure was low. The illustration below shows the measurements of energy intake and expenditure. There is an astonishing match between the two. Of course, these elite cyclists (and their support teams) know what they are doing. They know that they have to take in very large amounts of energy on the strenuous days. But the cyclists also rested when they could – not just rested physically, but also from the strain of eating so much during the race days. Therefore, these cyclists are not just professionals at expending energy, as we'd all imagine, but they are also elite eaters. Those who can't stomach 5,000–7,000 kcal/day aren't competitive.[7]

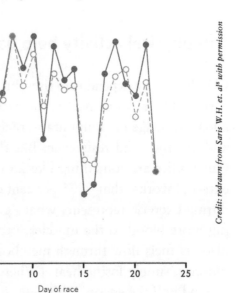

Credit: redrawn from Saris W.H. et al[8] with permission

Energy intake and expenditure in Tour de France cyclists. Solid points represent energy expenditure, open points energy intake. The low points on days 15 and 16, and also 22, represent rest days or shorter time trials. Typical energy intake for a young active adult would be around 2,900 kcal per day.

In each of these examples, we can see the energy balance model in action: and what we see is that these people are all expending so much energy that they may have difficulty taking in sufficient to maintain their body weight. Let nobody say that physical activity is not relevant to weight control – it all depends how much you do.

How, though, does that apply to the typical town dweller like myself, whose physical activity on many days isn't much more than getting to work and perhaps climbing some stairs, if there aren't too many, to our desk?

Can physical activity help balance our calories?

Clearly, energy expenditure rises during physical activity. Why is this? The obvious part is the external work done: pulling a loaded sledge up a mountain, racing a bike against gravity, and air and road resistance. But that's not the major part. Our bodies are something like 25 per cent efficient at doing external work – that is, 75 per cent of the energy expenditure during exercise represents what's going on inside us: pumping more blood to the muscles, breathing more deeply; and also, as fuels flow through metabolic pathways to drive our muscles, simply losing heat. (When we oxidise glucose, only around half the energy it liberates is transferred to ATP – described on page 74.) We therefore feel warm, and that's what Atwater was able to measure so easily in his calorimeter (explained in Chapter 2). Clearly, physical activity helps in terms of balancing our calories in and out. Why, then, is its role so often dismissed?

We often hear the numerical arguments against the usefulness of physical activity. Robert Lustig, in the much-viewed University of California YouTube video mentioned before,[9] dismisses it with the statement: 'you need twenty minutes of jogging to equal one chocolate chip cookie'. For a start, I think he underplays exercise: a quick literature search tells me that a typical chocolate chip cookie provides 80 kcal, whereas I calculate twenty minutes jogging at a reasonable pace (7.5 minutes/km) to use about 170 kcal, so I could eat two cookies and still be in balance. But, more seriously, this argument about how long it would take you to burn off any given snack isn't logical. One cookie, or even two, isn't going to change my weight much, but regular eating of such snacks may do. Similarly, I agree: one jog isn't going to change things much. But regular jogging, or any other form of exercise, is another matter. A typical figure is that jogging 1 km uses 62 kcal (more easily remembered as 1 mile of jogging uses 100 kcal). A casual jogger covering 20 km each week, a distance that serious runners would consider trivial, will therefore burn off 1,200 kcal (lots of cookies). My GPS watch tells me that I am such a jogger. Over the past twelve months, as a moderate-distance and slow-paced jogger going out two or three times a week for enjoyment, I have apparently burned 71,000 kcal while jogging. That's produced the same effect on my calorie balance as going for a month without food entirely. And I know which I prefer. As I write this, I've just come back from a jog, again with my friends Bobby and Alex. Admittedly, this was a rather hilly jog and longer than our usual, but my watch suggests that I used 1,100 kcal. If I were to eat a few chocolate-chip cookies now, I would still be in negative energy balance. But I won't, as my 'runners' high' helps me to resist the temptation to undo all the good – that flood of endorphins that makes you feel good after exercise.* 'I run so I can eat cake' is a slogan one sometimes sees in running magazines or on joggers' T-shirts. It seems perfectly justified.

There are various ways of looking at the energy cost of physical activity. Sport scientists might measure the oxygen consumption. But, more useful for most of us, is to know the energy used during various activities. Commonly, this is expressed in relation to an individual's resting energy expenditure, and the unit used is the MET (metabolic equivalent): 1 MET is the energy expenditure at rest; this falls to around 0.9 MET during sleep, and rises to around 3–4 MET for moderate

---

* 'Runners' high' has been investigated scientifically. It seems to consist of activation of both the endocannabinoid system (the internal system that is also activated by cannabis) and the endorphin system (the internal system activated by opium and related drugs). It dulls pain, produces euphoria, and is more marked after strenuous than light exercise.[10]

to brisk walking, 9 MET averaged over a day's hill-walking, 8–12 MET for jogging (depending on speed) and 18 MET for an elite marathon runner – but take all these as ball-park figures. (It's worth noting that the energy cost of jogging a fixed distance, say 1 km, does not depend on the speed: the faster runner will expend energy at a higher rate, but it will be over more quickly.) The energy costs of many activities have been collated by Barbara Ainsworth at Arizona State University and can be found online.[11] If you want to look at the effect on your own energy balance, strictly you need to remember that these are gross figures: if we weren't being physically active, we would still be expending 1 MET sitting down. But I would suggest that, as long as we're talking about moderately strenuous activities (say 5 MET or more), that's not really a big issue: the numbers are approximations anyway.

And indeed, many cross-sectional studies show that the more physically active people are, the less overweight they tend to be. In a pan-European study of 400,000 people, there were strong negative relationships between the level of physical activity and both BMI and waist circumference (that is, physical activity seemed to protect against these measures of obesity).[12] A similar relationship between physical activity and low BMI (and body fat) was seen in 250,000 people in the UK Biobank.[13] Loretta DiPietro at the Centers for Disease Control looked at this in 19,000 US adults. She found a clear inverse relationship between physical activity and body weight, with those reporting higher levels of physical activity less likely to be obese (BMI > 30 kg/m^2). Those who ran, jogged, performed aerobics or cycled weighed less, on average, than those reporting no physical activity. Walking came out as particularly protective against overweight in those above forty years of age.[14] In Colorado, a state with a low prevalence of obesity compared with the rest of the USA, a survey of walking showed that the more obese tended to walk less; and less walking correlated with more time sitting and watching television.[15] There are many similar studies on smaller numbers in different populations, albeit sometimes reporting relatively weak associations.

When it comes to specific forms of physical activity, there seems to be more in the literature on running than on other forms of physical activity (although, as a jogger myself, I admit to potential bias here). One example comes from the work of Stephen Blair at the University of South Carolina, an expert on physical activity. He is best known for his clear demonstrations that being fit overcomes many of the adverse health effects of being overweight – the 'fit fat' are relatively healthy (although, it should be said, also rather uncommon). In 2014 he published the results of a very large study, following 55,000 adults for fifteen years. Just under one-quarter of this American population jogged at all – some infrequently, others more regularly. There was a clear gradient of BMI across the groups, from non-joggers (highest BMI) to those jogging for three hours or more each week (lowest BMI).[16] Actually, the paper was aimed at determining effects on health, and the joggers had extremely clear advantages in terms of mortality from any cause. We'll come back to that later. Looking at other activities, cycling as a way of commuting (replacing car use) is strongly associated with a lower BMI, whereas in this particular study of 7,000 people, walking was not so.[17] Looking at 'Masters Athletes' (usually defined as more than thirty-five years in age), Walsh and colleagues in Australia found sixty individual studies, although numbers for each sport were small (for example, fourteen runners, four each of cyclists and soccer players, and three swimmers): runners indeed had the lowest BMI, although all athletes were leaner than non-athletic controls.[18]

We saw, in Chapter 7, that obesity has a strong genetic component. You might then ask, could exercise help someone who is genetically destined to put on weight? In a collaborative study between the Universidad Mayor, Santiago, Chile and the University of Glasgow, Carlos Celis-Morales and colleagues looked at how physical activity impacted upon people's genetic tendency to gain weight. They used data from 300,000 participants in the UK Biobank. They calculated a score for 'genetic risk for obesity' using genetic markers known to be linked to a tendency for obesity. Among those classed as 'inactive', the genetic risk score was strongly associated with their BMI; but this relationship was much weaker among the more active. Physical activity helped to overcome a genetic tendency to gain weight.[19]

Nevertheless, the relationships between physical activity and weight, while statistically significant, are not especially marked. In the pan-European study mentioned above, the average BMI of the least active compared with the most active was greater by 0.7 BMI units (kg/m^2). There are several obvious reasons why the relationship between regular physical activity and body weight might not be so strong as one could imagine. Of course, if we exercise more, we may want to eat more. The body's internal regulatory systems should see to that. The question is, whether we are tempted to under- or over-replace the energy we have expended on physical activity. My personal guess is that this very much depends on the circumstances. If I work out at our University's gym, there is a nice café where it just seems obvious I might go afterwards for a coffee and a snack. This is true of many commercial leisure centres, as they are now perversely called in the UK. Ron Maughan, an exercise physiologist in the UK, surveyed runners and showed that the greater the weekly running distance, the more the participants ate; but still, the more miles covered per week, the lower the body-fat content. The increased eating was not enough, in these runners, to offset all the increased energy expenditure.[20] A few studies suggest that those who exercise at higher intensities (for example, jogging versus walking) are slimmer, even when the total cost of exercise is similar. The explanation may be that the temptation to eat to replace calories lost is less after strenuous exercise – as my personal experience of runners' high might indicate.[21] Other studies show that regular exercisers may have similar body weight to more sedentary people, but they tend to have less body fat and more lean mass.[22] And, of course, if physical activity helps to maintain or increase lean body mass, this will in turn increase the resting energy expenditure, making it easier to balance the calories in and out.

Finally, I should mention that most of these studies are based on self-reported physical activity. We don't have so many studies of the reliability of this reporting, as we do for reporting of energy intake. What we have suggests that self-reporting generates rather random results.[23] But it would not be surprising if the less active might tend to over-report their physical activity, especially in view of all the public-health messages about this. And that would, again, dilute the results of cross-sectional studies. We should also note that physical activity doesn't have to be exercise: if we can simply accumulate activity in active travel to work, in gardening, in climbing stairs or dancing, we are less likely to feel a need to reward ourselves with a compensatory snack. It will all help to balance the calories in and out.

How much exercise do we need to shift our calorie balance?

If we measure someone's resting energy expenditure in the morning before breakfast, and extrapolate this over twenty-four hours, the number will be less than total energy expenditure measured with doubly labelled water. The difference between them represents several components, including postprandial thermogenesis (the extra heat released as a meal is digested and its nutrients stored), but the greatest difference comes from physical activity. The ratio of the two (total daily energy expenditure divided by resting energy expenditure extended over twenty-four hours) therefore broadly reflects the amount of physical activity, and is called the Physical Activity Level, PAL. It's a simple way of comparing different people's levels of activity – about as useful as is BMI for assessing fatness and thinness.

Klaas Westerterp, with John Speakman at the University of Aberdeen, tabulated the PAL in around 1,000 adults. PAL values around 1.5–1.7 were most common. Any value of PAL below 2.0 implies that resting energy expenditure accounts for more than half of total energy expenditure; so, clearly, for most people, resting energy expenditure dominates the total. Less than 15 per cent of people had PALs below 1.4, sometimes taken as the definition of being sedentary.[24] (Almost everyone will increase their energy expenditure simply by getting out of bed, moving around the house, washing, etc.)

In 2002 the first of a series of conferences held in honour of Mike Stock, the obesity expert we first met in Chapter 6, convened experts to discuss the requirements for physical activity. These experts reported that 'it seems likely that moderate intensity activity of approximately forty-five to sixty minutes per day, or 1.7 PAL is required to prevent the transition to overweight or obesity'. What does it take to achieve this? Let's just suppose, using very broad brushstrokes, that total daily energy expenditure is 2,500 kcal/day; then a sedentary person's PAL of 1.4 implies a physical activity-associated energy expenditure of 720 kcal/day, on top of 1,780 kcal/day of resting energy expenditure (so 2,500/1,780 = 1.4). To increase this PAL to 1.7, assuming resting energy expenditure remains unchanged, physical activity-associated energy expenditure would have to increase from 720 to 1,245 kcal/day: it would have to increase by 525 kcal/day, or 73 per cent. That would require something like fifty minutes of jogging each day, just as the Stock Conference experts concluded. These are not the levels of polar explorers, but they do require some sustained effort. The same experts suggested, though, that 'a good approach for many individuals to obtain the recommended level of physical activity is to reduce sedentary behaviour by incorporating more incidental and leisure-time activity into the daily routine' – it doesn't all have to be hard slog.[25]

How easy is it in practice to increase one's PAL? Westerterp reviewed ten studies of exercise interventions – encouraging people to increase their physical activity. In two studies the final PAL was greater than 2.0. These were in eleven-year-old and thirty-seven-year-old people. In the three studies he reviews in older people (average ages sixty-one, sixty-six and sixty-seven years) all showed initial PAL values below the value of 1.69 (indicating a 'light active lifestyle'), which failed to change with the intervention – bad news for my peers. Only one of the studies produced a loss in body weight, and that comprised 'the longest and possibly most demanding exercise training'. Thirty-two volunteers trained from an initial sedentary state to being able to run a half-marathon (21 kilometres). Nine of them dropped out, as it was too strenuous. And the average weight loss was just 1.0 kg. But there was a positive side: these volunteers lost fat, as expected, but gained fat-free mass, presumably largely muscle.[26] That will, of course, increase their resting energy expenditure.

All exercise is good for health, as we shall see shortly. And undoubtedly physical activity helps to keep the calories in and out balanced. But to expect physical activity alone to reduce body weight is asking a lot.

Physical activity as an aid to weight loss

In 1995 Andrew Prentice and Susan Jebb, both working then
at the UK Medical Research Council's Dunn Nutrition Unit
in Cambridge, published a paper titled 'Obesity in Britain:
Gluttony or sloth?'[27] They argued that the increase in obesity
could as well be due to low levels of physical activity (and
hence low energy expenditure) as to elevated levels of energy
intake. In support of their argument, they cited data that
seemed to show that, in the UK, energy consumption was
somewhat decreasing over the years, while levels of physical
inactivity were increasing. They chose as 'proxy markers' car
ownership and television viewing, and showed that increases
in these markers paralleled the increasing prevalence of obesity. It is certainly true that development of obesity requires an
energy imbalance that could, in principle, be due as much to
reduced expenditure as to increased intake, and it must be true
that physical inactivity will add to the 'Energy imbalance gap'
as described by Kevin Hall. I do think, though, as I explained
when we looked at obesity in the last chapter, that, on the
whole, lack of physical activity cannot be the main driver of
growing obesity rates.

The idea that increasing physical activity will aid weight
loss is an appealing one, however. Indeed, there are many,
many studies in which exercise has been added to diet for
the purposes of weight loss. The rationale is clear. Exercise
involves extra energy expenditure, so helping to tip the
person into negative energy balance (that is, losing weight).
With a restricted-energy diet, energy expenditure falls, as
it does during starvation. Exercise may help to keep energy
expenditure up. And what's more, enough exercise will, as
we saw with the half-marathon trainees, increase muscle (fat-
free mass), and so raise resting energy expenditure. And yet,

study after study finds that the result of adding exercise to a reduced-energy diet is not as great as hoped.

These studies were comprehensively reviewed for the Cochrane Database of Systematic Reviews by Kelly Shaw in Tasmania and colleagues. They looked at forty-three individual studies, involving nearly 3,500 participants. Exercise added to diet did help weight loss, but only to the tune of 1 kg extra. In studies in which diet and exercise were compared, the dieters always lost more weight (by about 4 kg) than the exercisers. The addition of exercise, though, was always beneficial in terms of improvement of cardiovascular risk markers such as reduction of blood pressure.[28]

There are various explanations as to why exercise doesn't aid weight loss as much as one might expect. Klaas Westerterp suggests some. He has produced evidence that one effect of physical training, in previously sedentary people, is to increase 'efficiency' of metabolism. Resting energy expenditure relates closely to fat-free mass, as we have seen, but with training the relationship changes so that there is somewhat less resting energy expenditure associated with each kg of fat-free mass. Westerterp also suggests that, at least in some people, increasing energy expenditure with exercise may lead to a compensatory decrease in other energy expenditure (for example, the non-exercise activity thermogenesis, NEAT – explained on page 120 – component: 'fidgeting').[29]

There has been clear evidence confirming this view in another group of people. The Hadza tribe of hunter-gatherers in Tanzania lead very active lifestyles. Herman Pontzer and colleagues at Hunter College, New York have studied these people in detail. The Hadzas appear to eat little, exercise a lot and maintain their weight at a lean level. This has led some to hypothesise that they have developed a very 'efficient' metabolism. But Pontzer and colleagues persuaded these people to have their total energy expenditure measured using the doubly labelled water technique, along with their resting energy expenditure. The Hadza men did indeed have a high PAL – average of 2.3. But their total daily energy expenditure was not different from westerners. The investigators concluded that the Hadza people compensate for their high energy expenditure in physical activity by reducing energy expended on their other activities.[30] As Pontzer puts it, 'We think the Hadzas' bodies have adjusted to the higher activity levels required for hunting and gathering by spending less energy elsewhere'[31] – perhaps by reducing non-exercise activity thermogenesis, NEAT. He has expanded on these arguments in his book *Burn: The Misunderstood Science of Metabolism*.

Dylan Thompson and his colleagues at the University of Bath have also looked at the reason that an exercise programme does not produce the weight loss one would expect from a calculation of the additional energy expended. In their study, however, they ruled out any compensatory drop in other forms of physical activity – they are experts at assessing all forms of physical activity using specialised sensors. In fact, they found evidence that a group of volunteers prescribed exercise sessions actually increased their non-exercise physical activity. But instead, Thompson and his colleagues found that the volunteers compensated for the increased energy expenditure by adding to their energy intake, to the extent of about 100 kcal per day. This was enough to convert an anticipated loss of weight of about 4 kg (based on the extra energy expended in activity) to an actual loss nearer to 1 kg.[32]

We therefore need sufficient exercise to exceed any compensation, whether that be from eating more or moving less outside the exercise sessions. As we saw earlier in this chapter, that might mean more exercise and at a higher intensity. That idea was tested by Kyle Flack at the University of Kentucky, who, with his colleagues, recruited a group of overweight or obese previously sedentary men and women. These volunteers followed a twelve-week protocol, exercising five days per week, at a level of either '300 kcal of exercise per session' or 600 kcal. That could mean, for example, in round figures thirty or sixty minutes of jogging per session. The higher-intensity group dropped their body weight and fat content, whereas the lower-intensity group did not, despite expending an extra 18,000 kcal above their baseline. The implication is that the higher-intensity group exceeded the threshold at which they could compensate for the additional expenditure.[33]

One related factor needs to be borne in mind. We have been looking at experimental settings in which participants have been prescribed exercise sessions, often conducted under supervision. If I were one of them, I daresay I would get home after the session and feel justified in putting my feet up for the rest of the day – in other words, the experimental design may be implicit in the disappointing result. To be anecdotal again, when I read my monthly running magazine, almost every issue has a story from someone who has slimmed down from being grossly overweight, and thanks running for helping them do so. Victor from Leeds, UK, is an example. At 165 kg he could barely breathe when walking, and knew he had to do something. With the help of Slimming World (and their low-fat diet) and picking up his running he lost 64 kg, dropped his waist size from 170 to 97 cm, and says, 'Running and weight loss go hand in hand. It's definitely helped with the weight loss – I know that for a fact.'* I am sure this is so: running – or any other form of exercise – can give such a positive mindset that it may help you to do all that's needed to lose weight (outside the strict confines of a controlled scientific experiment, that is). But still, these people must have reduced their energy intake as well as increasing their expenditure.

To be clear, then, if you want to lose weight, exercise will

---

* Quoted with Victor's permission.

help, but not perhaps as much as you might expect from the amount of energy expended – although it is possible that you are just not doing enough, or that you are compensating by resting outside the exercise sessions or sneaking extra snacks. But really, you will also need to focus on restricting what you eat. And, of course, I understand that there are those for whom all this talk of jogging sessions is inappropriate – many people physically cannot exercise at that level. In that case, you will have to rely on restricting the 'calories in' side of the equation in order to lose weight. We shall look at what the science tells us about how to do that in later chapters.

And for those wanting not to gain weight, there are clear benefits to keeping physical activity up: both in terms of helping to prevent weight gain, and in terms of benefits to health. The evidence is absolutely clear that exercise is good for everyone's metabolic health.

All exercise is good for you

All physical activity, whether or not structured as exercise, is good for you. There are endless scientific reports of the health benefits of being physically active. Several studies show that regular jogging will typically add five to six years of healthy life. And the same is true of other forms of exercise. Between 2010 and 2019 I chaired a Task Force for the British Nutrition Foundation (a non-governmental body giving advice on nutrition) to look at the evidence on nutrition and risk factors for cardiovascular disease (heart attacks and strokes). We looked at various dietary factors that could be beneficial. But a common thread running through our report, published in 2019, was the enormous power of exercise.[34] Better than any pill, and targeting so many different aspects of cardiovascular disease, exercise should be at the top of any doctor's treatment choices, especially in the context of disease prevention. And while physical activity is good for health, there is increasing evidence that the opposite is true: that long periods of remaining sedentary can outweigh these benefits. If I go for a run first thing in the morning, then spend the rest of the day sitting at my desk, I have probably undone the health benefits – although not necessarily the benefits to my calorie balance.

Many health authorities now endorse the view, summarised by the World Health Organization, that 'all adults should undertake 150–300 minutes of moderate-intensity, or 75–150 minutes of vigorous-intensity physical activity, or some equivalent combination of moderate-intensity and vigorous-intensity aerobic physical activity, per week'.[35] Being physically active helps with weight control, as we have seen, but it also helps protect against diabetes, cardiovascular disease, some forms of cancer, mental ill-health, dementia[36] and general ageing.[37]

Physical activity, calorie balance and health in perspective

The topic of physical activity and energy balance is a controversial one. We have seen conflicting views in this chapter. But, to summarise, we expend additional energy during physical activity. This must help us to balance our calories in and out. And yet exercise sometimes gets a bad press, for reasons that I think are often illogical. Physical activity alone, at the levels any of us might aspire to in our normal daily lives, is probably not enough to cause weight loss – for that, energy intake also has to be restricted. But for those who can manage regular strenuous exercise (such as jogging), exercise can certainly play an important role. And all physical activity is good for health and well-being.

We've now looked at calories in and out in a number of

settings. I hope I have been clear in saying that I believe the energy balance model – calories in–calories out – to be the principle that underlies our body-weight trajectory. But we have consistently seen just how easy it is to be misled about what any one person is eating, or how fast their metabolism – difficulties that I suspect are behind the issues that many people have with this model. Challenges to the energy balance model seem to be ever more prevalent.

9

A calorie is a calorie ... is a calorie: Challenges to the energy balance model

I was surprised to find, on a quick Internet search, that the cabbage-soup diet is still quite a big topic. Essentially, this promises that if you eat only cabbage soup for a week, you will lose 5–7 kg in weight. No surprise: it's almost devoid of calories.

No one, so far as I know, has suggested that this diet works by anything other than rebalancing the calories in and out. Your energy intake will fall to close to zero. Meanwhile, energy expenditure will continue, although it will fall somewhat because of the restricted energy intake. The body will dip into its fat reserves, having first depleted its glycogen and associated water – hence a large fall in weight (largely water) in the first week.

We have spent eight chapters looking at human energy balance. What I hope we have learned is that there are good reasons for thinking that this concept – that the balance between calories in and calories out determines our weight trajectory – holds for humans under many circumstances. But we've also seen how very easy it is to be misled about this. In particular, we've seen the difficulty of knowing just what any one person is eating, and how we all make judgements about metabolism from this potentially misleading information. When we bear this in mind, I feel we haven't yet had reason to doubt the energy balance principle. And yet that is just what is being suggested by many authorities, in the popular press and on social media, in books and even in the academic literature.

Arguments against the energy balance model: the hormone insulin as the villain

The recent story perhaps begins with US science journalist Gary Taubes's 2007 book *Good Calories: Bad Calories* (*The Diet Delusion* in the UK). So far as the academic literature goes, it begins with an essay by Taubes in the *British Medical Journal* in 2013.[1] This essay contains the essence of the argument that the energy balance model may be a misunderstanding of the cause of obesity. Taubes writes about two alternative hypotheses: the energy balance hypothesis, as I have described it in the preceding chapters, and the endocrinological (hormonal) hypothesis. The journal's own introduction says, 'The history of obesity research is a history of two competing hypotheses. Gary Taubes argues that the wrong hypothesis [the energy balance model] won out and that it is this hypothesis, along with substandard science, that has exacerbated the obesity crisis and the related chronic diseases.' Taubes reviews the history of research on the causes of obesity and how, when the hormone insulin was discovered, it was thought to be an essential part of the process. He goes on to suggest that carbohydrates, especially those that drive a rapid insulin response, are 'uniquely fattening' by driving fuel into storage as fat.

In Taubes's 2020 book *The Case for Keto* he asserts that:

If the conventional thinking and advice worked, if eating less and exercising more were a meaningful solution to the problem of obesity and excess weight, we wouldn't be here. If the true explanation for why we get fat were that we take in more calories than we expend and the excess is stored as fat, we wouldn't be here.[2]

There are some interesting claims in there that will take some unpacking.*

The 'insulin and obesity' argument is gathering momentum. Robert Lustig, the University of California paediatrician we have met a few times, describes in his book *Fat Chance: The Bitter Truth about Sugar* how 'In the body, insulin causes energy storage in fat cells ... Insulin delivers a one-two punch to drive gluttony and sloth, weight gain and obesity ... Insulin is the bad guy in this story.' And Jason Fung, a Canadian nephrologist and obesity specialist, in *The Obesity Code: Unlocking the Secrets of Weight Loss* describes the energy balance model (defined by him in a slightly restricted form, that 'Calories In–Calories Out = Body Fat') as 'the calorie deception'. 'Obesity', he says, 'is a hormonal, not a caloric, disorder.' He goes on to talk about the 'insulin causes obesity hypothesis' and cites many observations that appear to support it – observations we shall examine shortly.

These arguments crystallised during 2021/2022 with a series of exchanges in the *American Journal of Clinical Nutrition*. These began with the article that I mentioned in

---

* I don't want it to seem that I am picking on Taubes especially. He and I have talked about these issues; indeed, he quotes a conversation with me in *The Case for Keto*. But he's easy to cite because, as a journalist (his own description of himself), he writes very clearly – if not, in my opinion, correctly in this particular instance.

Chapter 1: David Ludwig, endocrinologist and Professor of Pediatrics at Harvard Medical School, together with a group of seventeen international and well-respected authorities in this field, claiming that 'obesity rates remain at historic highs, despite a persistent focus on eating less and moving more, as guided by the energy balance model (EBM). This public health failure may arise from a fundamental limitation of the EBM itself.'[3] This was followed by a riposte from an international group of obesity scientists, led by Kevin Hall whose work on obesity energetics we looked at in Chapter 7. There was then a response from Gary Taubes (a co-author on the Ludwig paper), then a further return from Hall and others.

Both sides in this correspondence seem to me to be muddying the water. The Hall group, although in principle saying something more like my own beliefs, introduce a description of the energy balance model that includes the biology of regulation of body weight (as in Chapter 5). This goes beyond how I have described the energy balance model in this book. (Indeed, it does not seem to include the rather obvious mechanism of awareness of the tightness of one's trouser belt.) To me, and I suspect to most readers, the ultimate question is whether it is indeed true that 'it all boils down to calories in–calories out': that energy balance, viewed in this way, is indeed the ultimate arbiter of our body-weight trajectory. I fully accept the challenge that, if that is true, how come decades of advice to eat less and exercise more have failed to prevent the rising tide of obesity? We will look at that. But I would rebut any challenge to that overall model.

We need, then, to understand exactly what those who are proposing alternative models are saying. And here, I have to admit, I struggle somewhat. In fact, in an earlier article Ludwig makes clear that he does not want to throw out the energy balance model. He says that 'like the Conventional Model [that I have called energy balance], CIM [the Carbohydrate-Insulin

Model] obeys the First Law of Thermodynamics specifying conservation of energy'. We can agree, then, that energy balance is an overriding principle. 'However,' he goes on to say, 'CIM considers overeating a consequence of increasing adiposity, not the primary cause.'[4] So now our disagreement seems to be over the reasons why many people find it difficult to eat appropriately to keep their weight steady. Elsewhere, though, a paper from Ludwig's colleagues states their belief that 'a high glycaemic load diet – by increasing insulin secretion – alters substrate partitioning toward fat deposition and promotes weight gain'.[5] That would seem to imply a belief that weight gain is a function of something more than just calorie excess. This model is expanded in places to suggest that, after insulin has packed away the nutrients in our cells, we are left with a fuel deficit in the bloodstream that may lead to increased hunger.[6] Other than in one limited sense, that I describe below, I don't see the evidence for this.

These different views of the regulation of body weight – the 'simple energy balance model' that I am arguing for, the more complex version including the biology of weight regulation, and the carbohydrate-insulin model – have been picked apart by the Harvard-based physician and researcher Jeffrey Flier. Flier asserts that the simple model is beyond argument, and then compares the carbohydrate-insulin model, CIM, with Hall's more complex energy balance model, EBM. As he says, neither model has yet satisfactorily explained the increasing prevalence of obesity, nor why some people are more susceptible than others. The intensity of the argument is illustrated by Flier thus: 'Many observers in the field who do not identify with either camp are surprised by the intensity of the debate, which from time to time goes beyond scientific discourse to include *ad hominem* exchanges. When it appears, that aspect of the CIM/EBM debate does nothing to enhance – and I think impairs – the scientific environment of obesity research.'[7]

It is certainly true that eating simple sugars can increase appetite in the short term. This is typically seen when someone takes a drink of pure glucose, say 75 grams. This was a standard way (now largely superseded) of testing for diabetes. The level of glucose in the blood will rise rapidly, leading to secretion of insulin, which sends the glucose speedily into the tissues, mainly muscle, and also stops the liver producing more glucose – all seemingly appropriate responses. But this can lead to a fall in the blood glucose to below the normal baseline level, and that fall may trigger a desire to eat more. We must see this as an unusual situation, which our metabolism has not evolved to deal with. Yes, hunter-gatherers will gorge on honey or fruit, but the sugar they contain is within a matrix of other substances that will slow its digestion, and also much will be fructose rather than glucose, which produces much less of an insulin response. They don't (or didn't) drink sugary fizzy drinks.

My main disagreement here is much more with the proposition, clearly stated by many, that obesity is a 'hormonal disorder'. There is no doubt that this can be true in some medical cases. Deficiency of thyroid hormone is one example. That is one state in which we can truly speak of 'slow metabolism'. The small number of people with genetic or acquired disorders in the appetite-regulation system – such as the very few who cannot make leptin, or those with brain injuries especially in the hypothalamus, as we saw in Chapter 5 – develop obesity, but not because of slow metabolism: because they have an enormous drive to eat. But in none of these cases is there anything to argue against the energy balance model. Most of these writers, though, are focusing on the hormone insulin.

As I have stated in several places, I have spent my career studying human metabolism and, inevitably, the hormone insulin has been a major focus of my research. For the past few decades my colleagues and I have, in particular, studied the role of insulin in regulating fat storage in our fat cells (adipocytes). I feel, then, that I have some qualifications to write about this issue.

Let's look at the idea that a hormonal issue underlies obesity, with a particular focus (in these writings) on the hormone insulin. Now, what is this supposed to explain? Is it meant to help explain the rapid increase in obesity that started in the second half of the last century? In that case it would be surprising if it's a genuine, intrinsic hormonal ab-normality – that just happens to have spread rapidly around the world, accompanying westernised lifestyles. But Ludwig and colleagues propose something different. They talk of 'the marked increase in GL across the population since the low-fat diet era – due to a concurrent increase in total carbohydrate and the exceptionally high GI of modern processed carbo-hydrates', where GL is glycaemic load, a description of how much carbohydrate has been eaten and how fast it raises the blood glucose level; GI, glycaemic index, measures how fast an individual carbohydrate source raises blood glucose. This doesn't seem the same as Taubes's argument of 'the alternative hypothesis that Newburgh's work had allegedly undermined was the idea that some intrinsic abnormality ... was at the root of the disorder. This was an endocrinological hypothe-sis.'[8] (Louis Newburgh was, Taubes claims, the originator in the 1920s of our present understanding of energy balance.)

My main issue here is that the genetic evidence about pro-pensity to obesity tells us overwhelmingly that the genes act through the pathways regulating appetite. There's very little evidence for a genetic signal influencing insulin secretion or, indeed, pathways of fat deposition. Ludwig cites a *Nature* paper from 2015 as showing genetic links between obesity and 'insulin secretion/action, energy metabolism, lipid biology and adipogenesis', but a careful reading of that paper makes it clear that overwhelmingly the genes whose functions we

understand involve pathways in the brain, and that some genetic signals that appear in pathways relating to insulin and its
action actually point in the *opposite* way to those that would
support the CIM.[9] There is also some genetic evidence from a
technique known as Mendelian randomisation. This approach
is based upon looking at large datasets in which the level of
insulin in the blood, taken thirty minutes after the volunteer
has drunk a solution of glucose, is measured. Genetic markers
that go with this 'trait' can then be identified. If these genetic
markers are then applied to another large set of people, we can
look to see whether those with genetically determined high insulin responses are, in fact, obese. There are three such studies
in the scientific literature. One looked only at the insulin level
after fasting overnight and found no relationship between genetic markers for that, and obesity. But more relevant are the
two that looked at the insulin response to glucose. One is from
Christina Astley in Boston and colleagues, including David
Ludwig. This showed the effect predicted by the authors:
genetic changes that went with raised insulin were also associated with obesity.[10] But it has to be noted that these genetic
studies, as we saw with obesity, only ever explain a small part
of the variability in anything. Later, in an independent study,
Anthony Nguyen from Toronto and colleagues refined this
study. They decided it would be more meaningful to look not
at 'raw' insulin levels, but to adjust them for the concurrent
glucose concentration. (Insulin responds to glucose. If people
vary, as they will, in blood-glucose level thirty minutes after
taking a glucose drink, we need to take that into account
when evaluating the insulin response.) These researchers again
found a relationship: genetic changes that went with higher
insulin responses were also related to higher BMI. But, oddly,
the type of increase in BMI that they found was not typical:
the insulin-genetic markers were associated with an increase
in leg fat, which may be relatively protective against metabolic

complications, and with changes in blood lipids that would be predicted to reduce the risk of heart disease.[11] It would be difficult to extrapolate from these studies to say that a high genetically determined insulin response is associated with common obesity.

Is insulin the driver of fat deposition rather than excess calories?

We need now to delve a little deeper into the role of insulin as a driver of fat deposition. Taubes writes of 'the identification of the hormone insulin in the early 1960s as the primary regulator of fat accumulation in fat cells'.[12] I agree, and some of that early work set the path of my own later research career. Our fat cells take up fat from the bloodstream in a process that is stimulated by insulin. But an equally important factor is the presence of dietary fat in the bloodstream as a milky emulsion (called chylomicrons – as the illustration 'The plasma (the watery part of the blood) turns milky when we eat fat' shows on page 68): this is the major, in fact, almost sole, substrate for fat deposition in our fat cells except under very unusual circumstances. It so happens that when we eat a meal that contains a mix of nutrients, we achieve a rise in insulin secretion (from carbohydrates and proteins in the meal), and the presence of dietary fat in the bloodstream ready to be taken up. But an equally important role for insulin is in regulating the process of fat mobilisation – releasing our stored fat for use in other tissues such as muscles, heart and liver. This process is strongly opposed by insulin. So, yes, insulin plays a major – in fact *the* major – role in regulating the amount of fat in our fat cells. Taubes in his book *The Case for Keto* uses a figure from my textbook on metabolism to illustrate this, highlighting in the text the many points where insulin acts.

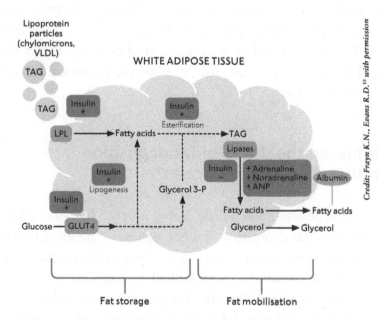

Diagram of the regulation of fat storage and mobilisation in adipose tissue, taken from my textbook *Human Metabolism: a Regulatory Perspective*, and reproduced by Gary Taubes in *The Case for Keto*. The figure shows the important – and complicated – role of insulin in regulating the amount of fat we have in our stores, but we interpret this differently. Taubes, and many others, suggest that insulin is the cause of excess fat deposition. I believe that insulin is the mediator by which changes in our energy balance are translated into the amount of fat we have in our stores. (Note that TAG is triacylglycerol, or fat.)

Here's the misunderstanding. Insulin can't drive net fat deposition (that is, the balance between fat storage and release) unless there's a substrate there for the process. We know that when there's a calorie excess, insulin levels will tend to rise, especially after meals; we know that the opposite is also true, insulin levels will fall when there's a calorie deficit. Insulin is then the mediator that adjusts the amount of fat in our fat cells to our state of energy balance – not the primary driver of how much we eat or store away.

Could insulin in itself drive fat deposition, without a calorie excess? Insulin is an anabolic hormone (it builds body tissues).

There are some striking pictures from the early 1920s, when insulin treatment was first introduced for the treatment of people with type-1 diabetes, that show emaciated figures transformed into healthy, even chubby youngsters.* There's no doubt that insulin played a part in allowing these youngsters to lay down both fat and protein. But you have to remember that before insulin came along, they were kept on almost starvation diets – the only way to prolong their lives. The insulin, when injected, also had something to work on, as they were allowed to eat more normally.

Recent loss of weight is one of the common presenting features of diabetes, type-1 or type-2, along with increased passing of urine and accompanying thirst. And when these patients are given insulin (or drugs with similar effects, for those with type-2) they will regain that weight. Insulin is being anabolic, yes. But the reason for their passing of urine is that the blood-glucose level is too high and glucose is spilling over into the urine, taking water with it. That represents a big loss of energy. As soon as that's stopped, by bringing the blood-glucose level back to more normal levels, that loss of energy in the urine is stopped. In the past few years, a new class of drug has been introduced for the treatment of type-2 diabetes. These drugs inhibit the mechanism by which the kidneys claim back the glucose from newly formed urine. The patient therefore goes back to peeing out glucose, which helps to lower the blood-glucose level. And, lo and behold, it turns out that these drugs also help to lower body weight. No surprise – they send calories down the pan.

The Diabetes Control and Complications Trial was a landmark American study of the treatment of type-1 diabetes that reported its results in 1993. It compared two types of treatment: the 'usual' standard of clinical care and insulin

---

* You can see one in *Understanding Human Metabolism* (CUP, 2022).

injections, and an intensive insulin group, whose insulin treatment was closely monitored and supervised to achieve much tighter control of blood glucose levels. The point of the study was to show that tight glucose control reduced the incidence of diabetes complications such as eye, kidney and nerve problems. (There have been similar studies since in type-2 diabetes.) But there were two major unwanted effects of intensive insulin treatment, one of which was weight gain.[14] Is that our proof? When we give extra insulin, does it indeed drive fat deposition? But the other side effect of intensive treatment was a considerably higher number of episodes of low blood glucose: hypoglycaemia. If you have ever experienced hypoglycaemia, you will know that it is a ferocious driver of appetite. I have been made hypoglycaemic (by insulin injection) on several occasions for experimental purposes. After one of these experiments I was offered a selection of sweet treats to help me recover. As I remember it, I stopped after my second Mars Bar, beginning to feel better at last. We don't have information on food intake among the DCCT participants, and anyway I am not sure it would be very useful given what we now know about food-intake records, but I would suggest that almost certainly the hypoglycaemia drove appetite, which led to weight gain. But there may be an even more important effect. A detailed study of the effect of intensive insulin treatment suggests that most of the weight gain was accounted for by eliminating glucose in the urine, with a smaller component representing decreased energy expenditure (it could well be that people with diabetes that is not under good control have increased energy expenditure).[15]

How about if we give extra insulin to laboratory animals, but stop them from eating more? Do they gain fat? Yes, there is some evidence for this, but the experiments are, to my mind, very artificial. In experiments in which insulin levels are raised in rats, they generally eat more and gain weight. But if they are not allowed any extra food, it is still possible to show a gain in fat. One such study is cited by Ludwig; but, in that experiment, body-weight gain was the same as in the non-insulin treated group. And you can bet that if those poor rats had been allowed access to extra food, they would have tucked in as though there's no tomorrow, and piled on the pounds (or grams, anyway).[16]

One final point against insulin as the primary driver of fat deposition is this. Suppose we had a medical way of increasing someone's insulin secretion. The CIM suggests that this would certainly lead to fat deposition. Oh, but we do. The drug semaglutide acts by mimicking the natural hormone called GLP-1 (described on page 102). GLP-1 is one of the hormones known as 'insulin secretagogues': hormones that increase insulin production after a meal. Semaglutide was developed for the treatment of type-2 diabetes, because it helps the patient produce more insulin. It's a very successful drug for that purpose (under the brand name Ozempic). And do these patients then get fat because they are making more insulin? No, they lose weight, and, as we saw earlier, semaglutide is now marketed for weight loss under the brand name Wegovy, and is touted for this purpose by a number of celebrities. The UK journalist David Aaronovitch has described his own experience with Wegovy. He says that he tends to become hypoglycaemic, and attributes this to 'eating less', forgetting, it seems, that semaglutide was developed to lower the blood glucose level.[17] And yet he has lost considerable weight. I just can't fit this into the CIM, although of course I have to admit that semaglutide might be a special case, as it also interferes with the pathways of appetite regulation that we looked at in Chapter 5. But as I write this, another drug is making the headlines for even more impressive weight-loss results in clinical trials. This is called tirzepatide and combines drugs that mimic the two human insulin secretagogues: GLP-1, as described above, and the other, called GIP (which stands for various things, but usually now glucose-dependent insulinotropic peptide). Both these components increase insulin secretion. Now, pharmaceutical companies are looking to target more receptors in this family. The story is interesting, because many people thought we would need to *block* these receptors to help weight loss. In fact, we need to activate them. And, oddly, the more you stimulate insulin secretion, the more it seems to reduce weight.[18]

Insulin, the mediator not the driver of weight gain – a recap

Let me summarise this long section about insulin and weight gain. Of course, insulin is involved in laying down fat. But I would say that insulin is the mediator between energy balance and our fat stores, not the primary driver. Questioning of the energy balance model and attempts to replace it with one based on insulin seems to start from the observation that we fail to change rising obesity levels by telling people to eat less and exercise more. But surely this is no surprise. Such regulatory systems as we have are now simply overwhelmed in today's environment. Arne Astrup, an internationally recognised nutrition and obesity researcher in Denmark, summarises it like this: 'We need to acknowledge that our regulatory systems are geared to prevent depletion of body energy stores and undernutrition effectively, whereas the systems that reduce appetite and increase energy expenditure during periods of excess availability of foods are easily suppressed by palatability and by the social, psychological, and rewarding aspects of foods.'[19] (It's just a bit surprising, then, that Astrup is one of the authors on the 2021 paper by Ludwig arguing against the energy balance model.)

I don't see evidence that insulin could be a primary driver of fat deposition, other than via increased energy intake. But this does seem a major argument of those proposing that we should all restrict our carbohydrate intake. But there is another aspect of their argument that we should examine closely.

How we lay down fat

When I started out in metabolic research, the pathways of fat metabolism were mostly understood in outline. But we didn't know how they operated in people going about their usual daily lives. It was clear that the pathway by which we can convert carbohydrates into fats for storage, *de novo* lipogenesis (described in Chapter 4 on page 81), was increased by insulin (in rodents). It made sense, then, to avoid eating carbohydrates, as they would stimulate insulin secretion, which would convert the sugars they contain into fat. But that's not what the science now says.

The notion that we should avoid carbohydrates, and sugars in particular, because they will be converted to fat and stored is a very popular one. A well-known UK physician explains: 'When you have more glucose than your body needs for energy, it eventually gets stored as body fat. This commonly happens when someone eats a high-carbohydrate (sugar & starch) diet.'[20] But it's not so. It is not a pathway by which we humans lay down fat except under exceptional circumstances. This was first shown by Reg Passmore, the Scottish physiologist whose work we examined in earlier chapters. Passmore started his paper with the words: 'Every woman knows that carbohydrate is fattening: this is a piece of common knowledge, which few nutritionists would dispute.'[21] He tested this by feeding volunteers large amounts of carbohydrates and looking at whether they were, indeed, converting these to fat.* What he found, in short, was that 'it is difficult to raise the RQ of man to 1.0 [this is the test of net fat synthesis], even when the subject undergoes real discomfort from his enforced gluttony'. Later, in the early 1980s, this phenomenon was investigated in detail by scientists at the Institute of Physiology in Lausanne. They found the same as Passmore: that a very large sugar-rich carbohydrate meal failed to switch the body to net fat synthesis. But they went on to show that this pathway, conversion of carbohydrate to fat, becomes important when someone is overfed (overfeeding, meaning feeding more than their energy requirement) with a carbohydrate-rich diet over a prolonged period. Under those conditions, the limited stores of glycogen in liver and muscle fill up, and the body's only way to dispose of excess carbohydrate is to store it as fat. But that is an extreme experimental situation, not one we would normally encounter.

The metabolic pathway for conversion of sugars into fats certainly operates in the human body, in the liver and to a limited extent in our fat cells, but under normal circumstances fat oxidation is greater than any fat synthesis. We lay down our fat stores by taking up dietary fat into the fat cells. We knew this anyway, because the pattern of fatty acids (monounsaturated, polyunsaturated, and so on) in our stored fat reflects our diet. As I described in Chapter 4, a modern understanding of the pathway for making fat from sugars is that it is important in regulating other pathways, in particular the oxidation of fat. Yes, lots of sugar will raise our fat stores, but this is because we encourage more dietary fat to go into storage and switch off mobilisation of the fat; not that the

---

* We can tell when the body is making fat in a net sense (i.e. synthesis is greater than oxidation) by looking at the ratio of carbon dioxide production to oxygen consumption, called the respiratory quotient or RQ.

sugar is directly converted into it. The fat stores are simply responding to energy balance.

We are trying to defend a weight set point that is too high

This idea of a set point for our weight, like a thermostat, is prevalent in the literature. Many people will seem to have a naturally stable weight and believe that this is intrinsically determined. But, as John Garrow pointed out, and indeed demonstrated by his personal experiments (see Chapter 5), it is difficult to demonstrate it. External cues (the reading on the bathroom scale) may be much more relevant.

One problem with the set point idea is that it would seem to override the principles of energy balance. Jason Fung in *The Obesity Code* writes that 'the problem in obesity is that the set point is too high'. He continues: 'A 30 per cent reduction in caloric intake results in a 30 per cent decrease in caloric expenditure. The end result is minimal weight loss.' This is plain wrong. The first part is correct: eventually the body will adjust energy expenditure to match intake, but that will be achieved by a considerable decrease in body weight. I tried simulating Fung's '30 per cent reduction in caloric intake' using the body-weight planner developed by Kevin Hall and others at the National Institutes of Health.[22] I suggested a starting weight of 85 kg and a desired weight of 60 kg to be reached in 365 days. The calculator says that my energy intake will have to fall by 24 per cent to maintain this 25 kg weight loss. I tried to get this to 30 per cent but the calculator told me that would involve reaching a dangerously low body weight.

It must be true that, for a fixed energy intake, our body weight will settle at a fixed point. As we saw in earlier chapters, when energy intake increases, so does expenditure, as lean body mass increases. And if intake decreases, so also does expenditure. They will find a point at which to settle. But that is not in any sense a set point. It is dependent on the balance between intake and expenditure and it is set by the calorie intake (and modified by the level of physical activity).

If there is, indeed, a set point for body weight, how would we show that? Presumably we would expect that when someone loses weight by reducing energy intake, their body will try to get back to its initial state. That person's body will behave differently from the body of someone who was naturally at this same low weight. Actually, the scientific evidence on this point is very mixed.

Some studies of people who have successfully slimmed down from being overweight show that they differ from people of the same weight who have never been obese. For example, studies headed by Catherine Geissler at King's College London looked at a group of 'post-obese' women compared with women who had never been obese. These scientists found consistently lower energy expenditure in the post-obese than in the never-obese women: 10–15 per cent lower resting energy expenditure, and lower expenditure following meals and during exercise.[23] Arne Astrup and colleagues in Copenhagen reviewed many studies and came to a similar conclusion.[24] But other investigators have not found this. A group based at the University of Alabama at Birmingham, USA, in collaboration with the Institute of Physiology in Lausanne, looked at twenty-four women who had slimmed down from an obese state, and compared them with twenty-four never-obese women. The women were matched for BMI, fat mass and fat-free mass. The investigators found no differences between the women in resting energy expenditure or postprandial thermogenesis.[25] Analyses of the post-obese women in the National Weight Control Registry database also found very similar body composition and energy expenditure compared with never-obese women.[26]

A possible reason for a difference in energy expenditure, where it's found, might be that people who have slimmed down from a greater weight have a different body composition (relative proportions of fat mass and fat-free mass) from the always-lean. But this is not found in the studies where it has been looked at. The evidence, as we saw in Chapter 6, does not support the idea that a low resting energy expenditure (or 'slow metabolism') normally underlies the tendency to become overweight. Perhaps, then, these post-obese people are still showing the lowering of energy expenditure that will have accompanied their energy restriction. One further factor might be that the post-obese have lower blood levels of leptin than the never-obese – and hence a greater drive to eat. This has been shown in several studies. Rudy Leibel at Columbia University, New York, who was involved in this field long before leptin was identified, has argued that this is one feature of the reduced-weight state that increases the propensity to regain weight.[27] Perhaps again this represents a carry-over, like the reduced energy expenditure, from the period when they were losing weight. These ideas have all been examined in depth by Catia Martins and colleagues at the Norwegian University of Science and Technology in Trondheim, together with scientists from the University of Alabama at Birmingham. Martins and colleagues suggest that the reduction in energy expenditure seen in people who have slimmed down may reflect on-going negative energy balance, and furthermore that even if a state of 'metabolic adaptation' to losing weight exists (meaning a long-standing reduction in energy expenditure), it is small, and bears no relationship to subsequent weight gain.[28]

Big fat confusion

'Wondering how to lose belly fat? This type of fat [mono-unsaturated] can also help prevent fat around the stomach area.'[29] 'Eating plenty of monounsaturated fats from avocados, olives and olive oil was also important for weight loss (on the low-carb diet).'[30]

What, then, is so special about these monounsaturated fats that they don't pile weight on, like other fats? As we saw in Chapter 4, there are different types of fatty acids: saturated and unsaturated. Among the latter are the monounsaturated, found especially in the foods listed above, and the polyunsaturated, typically prevalent in vegetable oils such as sunflower. To complicate matters further, polyunsaturated fats are further subdivided into families called n-6 and n-3, or, in popular literature, ω-6 and ω-3 (these are read as 'omega-6', and so on). I could write a book about fatty acids, their structures and their metabolism,* but suffice it to say for now that these different fats may be important for metabolic health, but the evidence that they contribute differently to calorie balance is limited and controversial.

There are, certainly, consistent reports of associations between different types of fat and body weight. A group from Laval University, Quebec, showed that reported intake of the different classes of fatty acids (I stress 'reported') was related to body weight: higher intake of saturated or monounsaturated fat went with more body fat, whereas for polyunsaturated fat there was no relationship.[31] In a similar study, but using markers in blood rather than dietary records, Michelle Micallef in Australia showed that high blood

---

* In fact I have, with colleagues: *Lipids: Biochemistry, Biotechnology and Health* (Gurr, M.I., et al., Wiley, 2016).

levels of *n*-3 (omega-3) fatty acids (which will have come mainly from fish) were associated with lower body weight.[32] But let's just remember all the potential confounders in this type of study: people who are better off, and especially those who are health conscious, are more likely than those less well-off to eat fish, avocados and olives, for example. Siôn Parry in Oxford, working with my colleague Leanne Hodson, showed that polyunsaturated fatty acids are more rapidly oxidised soon after a meal than are saturated,[33] but that does not mean that in the longer term they won't affect energy balance equally (if they are oxidised, something else is being spared).

Coming back to the study mentioned above from Éric Doucet at Laval, the overriding message from that study was that there was a strong relationship between *total* dietary fat intake (that is, irrespective of the type of fat) and adiposity.[34] Essentially, fat is fat when it comes to calories.

Efficient metabolism – the key to weight management?

Wouldn't you like to make your metabolism more efficient? This idea is often touted. For example, one UK celebrity physician who writes about matters of diet is quoted as saying that extending overnight fasting by not taking breakfast until 11am 'ramps up metabolism by enabling microbes to become more efficient at burning food'.[35] This is because:

> the microbes in our gut have a circadian rhythm like us and need a rest period ... Studies suggest a later breakfast to achieve 14 hours of fasting could help people to lose four to 11 pounds of weight [2–5 kg] over several months of doing it ... 14 hours of fasting overnight ... speeds up the

metabolism and helps people lose excess weight.[36] (These quotes are from newspaper reports.)

Clearly, then, we need to deal with our inefficient metabolism and our overworked, inefficient gut microbes, and speed up our metabolism (no need for exercise, though). But that's all a bit odd because, as I explained in Chapter 6, an 'efficient' metabolism is one that manages our energy budget very carefully and ensures that none is wasted – it's what we might call a 'slow metabolism'. No: what we want – if we think we can tinker with our metabolism to produce weight loss – is just the opposite: a very inefficient metabolism. And what do our gut microbes do that needs waking up? They work on food residues that arrive in the colon, breaking them down in a process called fermentation. These residues are known as dietary fibre, a broad term that includes a lot of carbohydrate-like substances that cannot be digested higher up the intestinal tract. The gut microbes act on this to make small molecules called volatile (or short-chain) fatty acids, that can then be used as an energy fuel by the cells of the colon and other tissues in the body. Make the gut microbes more efficient, and more energy will be rescued for the body, less will go down the pan: not quite what we are looking for.

My message is to watch out for metabolic black magic. It's unlikely to be based on science.

Energy balance is key despite many challenges

Despite all my objections to attempts to override the principle of energy balance, I do understand why so many are questioning how things can be so simple. All our attempts over several decades to halt the increasing prevalence of obesity by telling people to eat less and exercise more have been so spectacularly unsuccessful. My answer is to say that our present-day environment, which is changing all the time in a way that will drive energy surplus, is making it harder and harder for anyone to obey these apparently simple instructions. And metabolism works against us. It's incredibly difficult to lose weight (for good biological reasons), and, if we are successful, perhaps even more difficult to keep it off. And yet some people do manage just that, and we are fortunate that there is a good deal of research on exactly how they do it.

10

Why dieting is a struggle

Dieting challenges millions of years of our evolution. The last common ancestor of chimpanzees and humans lived 4–5 million years ago. Human evolution could be said to date from that time, in the Pliocene epoch, although many of our genetic characteristics must have been well established before that, since we share 99 per cent of our DNA sequence with chimps. But evolution has continued during much more recent times. Two examples stand out.

People living in societies in which starch is a major energy source have developed multiple copies of the gene that codes for the enzyme salivary amylase, important for digesting starch. We may have up to sixteen copies of this gene. In a study at the University of Sydney, local people had on average six copies, producing more amylase in their saliva; whereas chimpanzees have, and our even-closer relatives the Neanderthals had, just two (one on each chromosome).[1] Human populations who are not adapted to high-starch diets, such as rainforest hunter-gatherers and some fish-eating pastoralist societies, have a lower number of copies.[2] This development occurred somewhere in the last 200,000 years.[3]

An even more recent development is our ability to drink milk. Many of us take this for granted, but the milk produced by mammals evolved as nutrition for the newborn, not for the already well-nourished adult. Even now, in at least two-thirds of the human population, the gene that allows us to digest milk switches off after weaning.* So-called lactase persistence, which means adults can drink milk without unpleasant consequences, is present in populations in which dairying started perhaps 10,000 years ago. It is caused by a mutation in a gene that controls when the enzyme lactase is produced.[4]

We see that human evolution, in these cases aspects of our ability to benefit from different foods, has continued even over recent times. But one driving force for our evolution has undoubtedly been around for much longer: the threat of famine.

American nutritionist Ancel Keys, who conducted the Minnesota Study on partial starvation (mentioned in Chapter 2), thoroughly reviewed the known history of human famines in his account of that study, *The Biology of Human Starvation*. He listed and dated four hundred famines, but made clear that the list did not cover much of Asia (other than India) or the Americas, and was far from comprehensive. Andrew Prentice, whose work on obesity we looked at in Chapter 7, wrote movingly about human famines, drawing on his work in Africa.[5] Prentice asks us to consider that each one of us – anyone reading this page included – is the end-product of a line of people who have managed to survive whatever the world has thrown at them: famines among other

---

* The gene, called *LCT*, codes for the enzyme lactase, made in the small intestine, that breaks milk sugar, lactose, into its components: glucose and galactose. Those can then be taken up and used for energy. When the gene is switched off, lactose cannot be absorbed into the body and causes discomfort and diarrhoea.

hazards. There can be no doubt, therefore, that our ability to withstand times of food deprivation will be deeply embedded in our genetic make-up.

Prentice suggests the 'thrifty gene' hypothesis as a framework for understanding this aspect of our evolution. This hypothesis, first proposed by American geneticist James Neel in 1962,[6] suggests that those predisposed to developing diabetes are 'exceptionally efficient in the intake and/or utilization of food'. It has since then been adopted to cover the wider idea that we humans have thrived because of an innate ability to store away nutrients when available, and to live on remarkably little when needed. But this genotype has, as Neel put it, been 'rendered detrimental by progress'. There has been a lot of discussion about this idea in the intervening years, and it remains an ill-defined concept; it may cover many aspects of our metabolism and our behaviours. Still, it is difficult to get away from the fact that our bodies have evolved for far longer to withstand periods of famine than they have evolved to cope with nutritional plenty.

Of course, this is exactly what makes life so hard for many in the modern world. Our genes have been shaped to drive us to forage and gorge when we can, building up our stores; and when we wish to lose some of those stores, we are fighting against responses honed over many millions of years. John Garrow, who spent his career not just researching, but also treating, obesity, deliberately fattened himself up to see if he naturally returned to his former weight. He wrote: 'Since I am in the habit of telling obese patients that it is perfectly possible to reduce weight by 1 lb [1 pound, around 0.5 kg] per week by dietary restriction, I took my own advice and was gratified to find that it was true, although not as easy as I had expected.'[7] (Perhaps more physicians need to try the same thing.)

Our bodies are programmed to defend our fuel stores

You will have realised by now that this is not a diet book. There are too many of those already, in my opinion. And the very proliferation of diet books tells us that they are not really helping to solve the developed world's weight issues. Instead, I have chosen to write about the science behind weight issues, rather than giving you my personal opinion as to how to control your calorie balance. In so far as this book contains practical messages, they are more about how to avoid piling on the pounds. But, of course, many people reading this will be interested in losing some of those pounds. (A YouGov survey suggests that more than half the world's population is trying to lose weight at any one time.[8]) Of course, you will know already that losing pounds is going to be hard, partly for the reasons I've just outlined. But, despite that bad news, there are indications of how to make it less hard.

Dieting of necessity involves putting the body into a state of partial starvation – or, as I would put it, negative energy balance, changing the balance of calories in and out. In principle we might tip energy balance in the desired direction by increasing the expenditure side, but, as we saw in Chapter 8, you probably need to trek to the South Pole dragging a sledge to make this work unless you also cut down on calorie intake. But both increased physical activity and decreasing intake can play a role.

There is a vast scientific literature about just how the body responds to a state of negative energy balance: partial or total starvation. I reviewed briefly at the end of Chapter 2 how our fuel stores respond to energy deprivation. We quickly lose our relatively heavy glycogen, with its associated water, before beginning to draw on our (more considerable) fat stores.

We store our surplus energy mostly as fat for a good reason: it's a very energy-dense form of storage. What that means is that for each kilocalorie that we draw out of the stores, our weight isn't going to change much. Suppose we create a daily energy deficit of 1,000 kcal. If this is taken from the store of glycogen (with water), it will represent a drop in weight of 1 kilogram, whereas if this comes from the fat stores, the drop will be a mere 100 grams. And, as I noted in Chapter 2, any transgression will put back the glycogen and water, to the great dismay of the dieter.

That's not all that works against us. A consistent feature of lowering energy intake is that the rate of energy expenditure (the 'metabolic rate') falls. It's a powerful mechanism to protect us from the effects of starvation. That means you have not just to reduce the 'calories in' below what they were, you've got to reduce them even further because of the fall in energy expenditure. That's why there are so many diets and diet books. People have become rich because of the difficulty of dieting.

Francis Benedict at the University of Connecticut, who worked with Wilbur Atwater on the early human calorimetry studies, is equally well known for his study of human starvation. Benedict recruited a Maltese lawyer, Agostino Levanzin, as an experimental subject. Levanzin fasted for 31 days, mostly while living in the Atwater-Benedict calorimeter. His body weight fell from 61 to 47 kg (he started the fast in quite a thin state). Benedict noted that the rate of weight loss was greatest during the first few days, as glycogen was used up and water was lost from the body. Levanzin's energy expenditure, measured in the calorimeter, fell from about 1,500 kcal/day to 1,100 kcal/day. Benedict's long report of these studies, 'A study of prolonged fasting', was published in 1915.[9] It led to our understanding that lowering of energy expenditure during fasting is part of the body's adaptation to a lack of food, enabling it to keep going for longer with its limited reserves.

Our most detailed understanding of this response comes from Ancel Keys' Minnesota Study of semi-starvation, conducted with Conscientious Objectors in 1944/5. Thirty-two men were recruited for the study. Their baseline diet of 3,200 kcal/day was cut to 1,570 kcal/day during twenty-four weeks of semi-starvation. The men lost 16 kg in weight on average. Resting energy expenditure – or 'basal metabolic rate', as Keys called it (expressed for the whole person), fell gradually, to around 60 per cent of the initial value. Keys recognised that this arose partly because the men had lost body mass, so he expressed the energy expenditure in relation to body surface area (calculated by a formula – surface area is sometimes taken to represent the active tissue mass): it fell to 68 per cent of the initial value. He also calculated what he referred to as 'active tissue mass', meaning essentially all the body other than bones, fat and water compartments. Resting energy expenditure when expressed in this way fell by 16 per cent. It was therefore clear that the fall in energy expenditure reflected something more than the loss of body mass. Keys speculated on what might bring this about (he did not have the ability to measure concentrations of relevant hormones, such as thyroid hormone, in blood): he thought the heart was working less hard as the men lost weight (heart rate dropped from 55 to 35 beats/minute), that their muscles lost 'tone', and he noted a small drop in body temperature, which would reduce the rate of metabolic reactions.[10]

We see this very clearly in studies of people attempting to lose weight by restricting energy intake. For example, Rudy Leibel and colleagues at Rockefeller University in New York measured energy expenditure in a group of obese people who lost 10 per cent of their body weight on an 800 kcal/day diet. Energy expenditure went from 3,100 kcal/day to 2,550 kcal/

day, and, again, this was more than would have been predicted from the fall in fat-free mass. In another group, who
lost 20 per cent of their body weight, energy expenditure fell
even further, by 890 kcal/day. In a sub-group who then returned to their original weight, energy expenditure returned
to exactly where it had been before.[11]

We now know at least part of the mechanism involved in reduced energy expenditure with weight loss. One major factor
regulating energy expenditure, irrespective of body weight, is
the secretion of thyroid hormone. Thyroid hormone, which
is a modified amino acid liberated from the thyroid gland in
the neck, stimulates cellular energy expenditure by means
which are still not entirely understood despite more than 100
years elapsing since its discovery on Christmas Day in 1914.
Thyroid hormone concentrations fall when energy intake is
reduced, and there is now reasonably consistent evidence that
this is brought about by a fall in leptin concentration in the
blood. That would point once again to leptin, the sensor of fat
stores, as a key regulator of energy balance (as explained on
page 93–8 of Chapter 5). The leptin concentration in blood is
mainly a long-term reflection of the body's fat stores. But to
some extent it also reflects the current state of energy balance
(positive: gaining weight; or negative: losing weight). This has
been shown much more clearly in human experiments than
in mice, not least because it's so much easier to take regular
blood samples and to persuade the experimental subjects to
eat, or not eat, as required for the experiment. Blood leptin
concentration may fall by more than 50 per cent when people
fast for just a few days, losing only a small percentage (less
than 4 per cent) of their body weight, reflecting the energy
deficit.[12] Equally, a small increase in energy intake will raise
leptin without changing body weight.

Which diet to choose?

A close relative of mine has recently lost weight dramatically through a National Health Service referral to a commercial organisation – like Victor, the formerly overweight runner we met in Chapter 8. Their diet plan emphasises reduction in fat intake. (That agrees with one of my own strategies, developed when I was much younger, to keep my weight steady: giving up as much fat as I could, for example by not spreading margarine or butter on my toast, just putting the marmalade straight on.) Other, even closer relatives, swear by restriction of carbohydrates (they would have the butter but not the toast or the marmalade). Good friends follow a 5:2 diet with reduced intake on two days each week. And an academic collaborator lost considerable weight simply by taking smaller portions, and if his portion seemed larger than he needed, leaving part of it on his plate.

This is all anecdotal, however. And the problem with diet plans is that most of them are based on anecdote. Here I'm going to describe what we know – what has been shown in a scientific way – to help weight loss. I will point out now that this is, in some ways, straightforward – at least in theory. Any plan that cuts your calorie intake, and preferably also increases calorie expenditure, will work in due course. What is more challenging is the longer-term goal of maintaining that weight loss. We will come to that later.

In the 1960s, physicians in Boston, USA, led by George Cahill, treated obesity by what was euphemistically called 'therapeutic starvation' (actually it really was starvation, save for water, vitamins and minerals). Unsurprisingly, the patients, who were kept in hospital under observation, lost weight at a steady rate. These patients formed the material for a number of research studies on how the body adapts to starvation. We

know, for example, that ketone bodies can be a major fuel for
the brain during starvation (mentioned in Chapter 4) through
measurements made on some of these starving patients. In
other American centres, there are records of patients being
starved for long periods: in one case, a graph in a research
paper shows a patient who weighed 170 kg initially, ending up
after nineteen weeks at 110 kg.[13] (We are used to thinking of
obesity as a condition that may lead to many adverse health
issues – but when famine comes, those with extra weight will
be laughing at the skinny ones.) But this trend was taken to
extremes. In a study from Southampton, UK, obese patients
fasted for up to forty-five weeks. Two of the seven patients
lost more than half their initial body weight. Losses of lean
tissue (fat-free mass) were considerable, to dangerously low
levels. Indeed, one patient, a 19-year-old girl, died early in the
refeeding period after starving for 33 weeks, during which
she lost almost half her body weight.[14]

An alternative to complete fasting is to drastically reduce
calorie intake using a proprietary very low-calorie diet,
technically a liquid-formula diet, usually described as 'soup
and shakes'. Typically, this provides around 800 kcal per
day. This was first widely commercialised by Alan Howard,
a Cambridge scientist, as The Cambridge Diet in 1984.
In the UK, soup-and-shake diets have been used for rapid
weight loss in people with type-2 diabetes. The Diabetes
Remission Clinical Trial (DiRECT) helps people to lose
weight rapidly on an 800 kcal per day diet. It has shown
remarkable results in terms of putting the diabetes into remission for at least five years in some people.*[15] (Roy Taylor,
the instigator, believes this is because the rapid weight loss
removes fat from organs such as the liver and pancreas.[16])

---

* It was already known that rapid weight loss brought about by bariatric
surgery – stomach stapling and the like – could reverse type-2 diabetes.

One concern with drastic calorie reduction has always been the loss of body protein. If protein is lost, that comes from the fat-free mass, mainly the muscles. And, as we have seen in earlier chapters, fat-free mass is the main determinant of resting energy expenditure. A fall in fat-free mass will therefore lead to a fall in energy expenditure, as well, potentially, as limiting the dieter's ability to do (or enjoy) exercise. In the 1970s, Bruce Bistrian, a Boston, USA physician, promoted what he called the Protein-Sparing Modified Fast, described by him as a 'semistarvation regimen'.[17] Key features were the absence of carbohydrate but a supply of good-quality (animal-derived) protein and appropriate minerals needed for lean tissue retention. It was claimed that 'exercise tolerance is increased during weight loss in untrained subjects'.

To be clear, however, these soup-and-shake diets may help you to lose excess weight, but they are not a way to maintain that weight loss in the long term. For that, a transition to a conventional food-based way of eating is needed. This issue has been addressed in the DiRECT trial. The investigators, led by Mike Lean in Glasgow, have invested a lot of effort into managing a transition phase from severe calorie restriction to long-term weight maintenance. The transition phase lasts from around week twelve to week eighteen, and then a fully food-based dietary plan is followed, together with an increase in physical activity for those who can. Probably most importantly, the participants have intensive individual support.[18] Of course, most of us cannot have that level of support, and this is where the real difficulties arise.

Given that, it might be preferable to manage the weight-loss phase by eating real foods rather than synthetic concoctions. You probably feel you eat real food already, so how will that help? You have to find a way to take in fewer calories. Naturally, what most of us want is to be able to eat what we like and still somehow lose weight. But the history of dieting shows that there is no such magic transformation of our diet – if there were, we wouldn't be where we are. It will be difficult, and it will involve changes.

There are many options to choose from: low-fat, low-carbohydrate, smaller portion sizes, time-restricted eating, intermittent fasting – they are all ways of reducing energy intake, that work for some people.* Unfortunately, the very popularity of all these ways of losing weight hints at the problem: even if you manage it, the chances are you will be trying again after a year or two. It's a bit like the old joke, 'It's very easy to quit smoking – I've done it lots of times.' However, there is some research to guide you. There are research papers showing advantages to low-fat diets and there are papers favouring low-carbohydrate diets. I found four meta-analyses (combining results from different studies) comparing these diets for weight loss over periods of up to two years. They all find that, on average, those on low-carbohydrate diets tend to lose somewhat more weight than those on low-fat diets,[19] although the longer the duration of the diet, the less difference is seen.[20] So my simple, admittedly unscientific, meta-analysis of meta-analyses would suggest that the low-carbohydrate diet may be a better option, at least in the short term. A small study from Oxford suggests that it's quite possible to devise a food-based low-carbohydrate diet with similar energy to the 'soup-and-shake' diets (800–1,000 kcal/day), which leads to good weight loss (7.5 kg more than a control group) over twelve weeks.[21] But please note that this doesn't change my opinion at all about the underlying basis for weight gain or loss.

---

* Giles Yeo has addressed many of these in his book *Why Calories Don't Count*, showing how each works by restricting calorie intake.

Cut the carbs

American cardiologist Robert Atkins published his book *Dr Atkins' Diet Revolution* (later republished as *Dr Atkins' New Diet Revolution*) in 1972, which first promoted to the general public the idea that restricting dietary carbohydrate intake was the key to losing weight. It became the bestselling diet book of all time and was among the top fifty bestselling books in history. Atkins is said to have told people to 'eat the hamburger and throw away the bun'.[22] Since that time, many variations on the theme have been promoted, with differences in the level of restriction on carbohydrate intake, and what else you can or cannot eat. These include the popular 'Paleo diet', the 'South Beach diet' and the 'keto diet'. There are websites that review all these different options.[23] The keto diet involves very strict reduction of carbohydrate intake, to less than 50 grams per day: some 'experts' recommend going as low as 30 or even 20 grams per day. It is claimed that 6 per cent of Americans (15.5 million) are following this extreme version each year.[24]

Whether this is a good way to keep weight off in the long term, and whether it's good for your health, are much discussed. Many people interpret a low-carbohydrate diet to mean that they may indulge themselves in fatty foods such as cheaper or processed meats (such as burgers). This worries nutritionists, as it means a large intake of saturated fats, and indeed there are now many studies, and meta-analyses of multiple studies, that link consumption of low-carbohydrate diets to increased mortality, mainly from cardiovascular disease.[25] One large study with detailed records of food intake concluded that 'mortality increased when carbohydrates were exchanged for animal-derived fat or protein, and ... decreased when the substitutions were plant-based'.[26] Although more research is needed on these associations, I stress here that we are discussing these diets as a means of achieving weight loss, not necessarily of keeping weight off in the longer term: that we will look at in the next chapter.

Here I want to consider the many claims that these low-carbohydrate diets work through a metabolic or hormonal mechanism. To quote Taubes again: 'carbohydrate-rich foods create a hormonal milieu in the human body that works to trap calories as fat rather than burn them for fuel'.[27] My argument, in contrast, is that we should not confuse this with anything other than a straightforward application of the energy balance model. In the average American diet, taking figures from the US National Health and Nutrition Examination Survey (NHANES), carbohydrates supply 47 per cent of energy, with 22 per cent of that coming from added sugars. (This will include data from all those following low-carbohydrate diets, so the contribution of carbohydrates to energy for the average non-dieting American will be even higher.) In the UK the latest data from the National Diet and Nutrition Survey (NDNS) show 45 per cent of energy from carbohydrates.[28] If the aspiring dieter removes most of this energy, it would require a big increase in fat and pro-tein intake to get back those calories. A review of published studies has confirmed that low-carbohydrate diets help with weight loss because of reduced calorie intake rather than any specific effects of the lowering of carbohydrates.[29]

There is some research that helps us understand why low-carbohydrate diets help many people to lose weight. A feature of keeping carbohydrate intake (especially refined carbohydrates and sugars) low is that insulin levels remain suppressed. And that will encourage the production of ketone bodies from fatty acids. I explained in Chapter 4 that ketone bodies are a water-soluble product of fatty acid breakdown, which can be used as a fuel by many tissues including the brain. They are a means of ensuring the brain (which cannot extract fatty acids from the blood) gets sufficient fuel when its usual fuel, glucose, is in short supply. There is reasonably strong evidence that high levels of ketone bodies suppress appetite.[30] It is said that people who fast completely don't feel great hunger, whereas the volunteers in the Minnesota Study of partial starvation were ravenously hungry, and indeed some were rejected because they sneaked out to get extra food. Clearly this will help the dieter to stick to the plan. If carbohydrates are replaced mainly with protein, there are other potential benefits. Among the nutrients in our diet, protein has the best satiating power: it keeps our desire to eat again low for longer than do carbohydrate or fat.[31] Tucking into a meal rich in lean meat, for example, may help you to reduce calorie intake, because it will prolong the period before you want to eat again. In addition, protein has the largest effect on postprandial thermogenesis.[32] Postprandial thermogenesis, also called diet-induced thermogenesis, refers to the increase in energy expenditure (thermogenesis) that always occurs after a meal (the postprandial period). It is attributed to the energetic costs of digestion (moving substances through the digestive tract), transport of nutrients around the bloodstream and storing them in cells. (We looked at it briefly in Chapter 6 in connection with fast and slow metabolism.) Postprandial thermogenesis is one of the components of our 24-hour energy expenditure. Resting energy expenditure is usually the biggest, as we saw in Chapter 8 when considering physical activity. Physical activity-related energy expenditure is next, even for the sedentary, and postprandial thermogenesis typically accounts for at most 10 per cent of the total. Increasing this slightly by substituting protein for carbohydrate will help, although it is a small effect.[33]

There are also suggestions that low-carbohydrate diets,

especially the extreme variety, ketogenic diets,* increase energy expenditure compared with low-fat diets. The evidence on this point is not completely consistent, and it seems to depend on the duration of the diet, but overall it tends to support this idea.[34] It may not be a big effect, but every little helps. But whatever the effects of the protein content of a low-carbohydrate diet on satiety or thermogenesis, still these are not contradicting the principles of the energy balance model.

Keeping active

In Chapter 8 we saw that adding physical activity to calorie restriction doesn't, in most controlled trials, help the weight loss as much as we might expect, or hope. But that should not be a reason for staying sedentary. As I explained, the design of those experiments may work against the idea that weight loss will be helped by increasing activity. There are plenty of anecdotes of people who claim that exercise helped them to change their relationship with food. Jim Hill and Holly Wyatt address this issue in their book *The State of Slim*, based on their experiences studying Coloradans, who are generally slimmer than other Americans. They describe how 'losing weight without increasing physical activity makes it practically impossible to relax your diet vigilance even a little', and call exercise 'your Drano' (a proprietary drain-cleaning product – the idea is to open up your drain; that is, ability to burn off calories). And despite the somewhat negative message you may have picked up from Chapter 8, I should stress that no scientific study has shown increased physical activity to

---

* It should be noted that ketogenic diets are not new. They were introduced in the 1920s for the treatment of epilepsy (presumably the brain's electrical activity is more stable when fuelled by ketone bodies), and they need not be weight-losing.[35]

make weight loss *more* difficult: in almost all it helps, just not as much as the calculations might predict.

The literature on losing weight, however, also tells us that the difficulty doesn't stop with losing it. In some ways, it only starts there. The big issue is then keeping it off.

So you've lost some weight – what now?

There are various theories as to why maintaining weight loss is so very difficult, some of which I covered in the last chapter. It could be that by the time you reach your target weight, your energy expenditure has fallen, and it will seem that you need to eat even less than your friend who never put on weight in the first place. Whether this is really true after your weight has stabilised is not clear (we looked at that issue in the previous chapter). But the data are unequivocal. By whatever means people lose weight, it tends then to go back on. A long-term study using NHANES data in the USA showed that one in six adults who had been overweight had managed to sustain weight loss of at least 10 per cent. That means that more than 80 per cent who manage to lose weight put it back on.[36] Those figures should not deter you from trying. A large-scale review of weight-loss programmes showed that it takes around five years for the weight to go back on, and during that time risk factors for various diseases are all improved, with some evidence that there are long-term health gains.[37]

If you want to keep the weight off, you're going to need to change your way of eating and probably other aspects of your life. What works during a phase of weight loss may not be what you can stick with for the rest of your life (and, as I mentioned earlier, it might not be good for your health). But there are many scientific studies that tell us about how the successful 'weight loss maintainers' manage this.

We can get an idea of what is required from the National Weight Control Registry, run by Brown University and the University of Colorado, a database of people in the USA who have successfully maintained weight loss for at least one year.[38] On average, members of the register have lost 30 kg and kept that off for 5.5 years. Many report that keeping the weight off has been harder than losing it in the first place, but the good news is that keeping it off becomes easier with time. Those who maintain the weight loss for two years or more have a greatly increased chance of keeping it off in the long term.[39]

On average, the registry members follow a diet that is low in fat (average 24 per cent energy from fat),[40] they are physically active (doing around 1 hour per day of exercise)[41] and watch less television than the average American,[42] they mostly eat breakfast, and, interestingly, the more often they weigh themselves, the higher their chance of success.[43] Data from the UK's DiRECT Study bear out the importance of physical activity: participants who managed to maintain more than 10 per cent weight loss were more physically active, and had fewer periods of inactivity, than those who did not.[44]

Broadening this out, there have been several meta-analyses of the determinants of successful weight-loss maintenance. One of the most recent and comprehensive, by Rita Varkevisser and colleagues in Amsterdam, surveyed 67 articles on weight loss and extracted the characteristics of successful maintainers. Weighing regularly, control of portion sizes, an increase in fruit and vegetable consumption, reduction in dietary fat and in sugar-sweetened beverages, together with increased physical activity, were all strongly predictive of successful weight loss maintenance.[45] These characteristics are found in almost all studies. In Chapter 8 we looked at the rather negative views that many people have of the role of physical activity in balancing the calories in and out, but it shines through here as a consistent factor in helping people to maintain weight loss.

Jim Hill and his colleagues examined this, and they propose that an increase in physical activity is the only way for people to maintain weight loss in today's environment of high calorie availability.[46]

These data have given me pause for thought. There is no doubt that it is hard for someone who has successfully lost weight to keep it off. The scales seem tipped against them, so I thought I would look at the scientific literature to see just what someone who has never gained weight in the first place does. But I don't find much. There are some data from the National Weight Control Registry comparing successful weight losers with 'normal controls' – people with no history of overweight. The weight-loss maintainers do more moderate-to-vigorous physical activity than do the controls, but both groups do more than a currently obese group; and sedentary time is low in both the 'maintainers' and the controls compared with the currently obese.[47]

To my surprise, however, little seems to be known about what the 'never-overweight' eat. It seems a study that is crying out to be done. In the National Weight Control Registry, the weight-loss maintainers have greater total daily energy expenditure (measured with doubly labelled water) than the never-overweight (average 2,500 kcal compared with 2,200 kcal).[48] That might suggest that those who never gain weight eat less than successful weight-loss maintainers, but the latter group compensate by increasing moderate-to-vigorous physical activity; however, I think we need to see more research on this. The maintainers' daily energy expenditure was similar to that of an obese group (2,600 kcal), suggesting that they had hardly altered their energy intake from their former obese state. That seems unlikely, especially in view of some data (reviewed under my explanation of 'set point' on page 187 in Chapter 9) suggesting that those who lose weight have lower energy expenditure than those who were never obese.

Losing weight and keeping it off – a challenge in today's world

We all face difficulties in managing our calorie balance in to-day's world of plentiful calories and labour-saving devices. Of course, some people, because of their genes and other factors, are challenged more than others. Still, there are lessons for all in the research on people who have successfully lost weight, and especially those who have kept it off. But how about those who haven't especially put on excess, and want to keep it that way? There is a vast body of scientific evidence about aspects of our diet and our tendency to put on, or not put on, weight. Perhaps surprisingly, it's not all about cutting down what we eat – it's much more about eating those things that won't give us too many calories but will still fill us up (and be tempting and tasty).

11

Evidence-based eating

I've left home in a hurry – no time to make my lunchtime sandwiches, which I would normally eat with an apple or banana. I call in at the supermarket to buy some. Oh, but there's a 'meal deal' on offer for not much more, so I may as well get a snack – perhaps a bag of crisps today, or shall I go for a chocolate bar? – and a drink. (I could choose the water, but what's the point in paying for that? So I'll go for something sweeter.)

And somehow now I've worked too late to come home and cook dinner, so I'll just pick something up on the way home. There's an array of take-away food outlets to choose from, all providing tasty, convenient food in portion sizes that I know will fill me up – I just need to pop them in the microwave.

These scenarios are probably familiar to many. This is just to emphasise how we are surrounded by tempting calories and by things about whose composition we have little, if any, idea. Trying to balance your calories in and out has never been harder (except, perhaps, for many of our ancestors, who will have struggled to get enough on the 'calories in' side).

We have looked at how some of those who have shed unwanted pounds manage to maintain their weight loss. But we also know a lot about the foods that help people to keep a steady weight among all these goodies. In fact, those two strands will lead us to similar conclusions.

What exactly should we be eating?
The idea of energy density

Now I've made some time to cook properly. I bought a selection of root vegetables at the market, so I'll make a big pot of tasty vegetable stew, to which I'll add some lentils or perhaps chickpeas. And while that's cooking, I'll put some potatoes in the oven to bake – in their skins, of course, and I'll cook some green vegetables to go with them.

Perhaps, after all, I can't be bothered. I need to respond to some messages on my phone, so I'll get a pizza out of the freezer and eat that instead. I offer the thought that with the first meal I might struggle to eat the calories that I need, whereas with the second, it's all too easy.

Lauren Lissner at Cornell University, New York, wanted to test the idea that if you load more calories into a given amount of food, people will then eat more. She and her colleagues devised foods of low-, medium- and high-fat content. Calories went the same way. Protein was constant, so carbohydrate varied in the opposite way to fat; for example, the experimenters made three varieties of blueberry muffin, varying the amount of vegetable oil used. The volunteers, twenty-four women, followed each diet for seven days. The results were clear. The participants tended to eat about the same amount of food each day (1,400 to 1,500 grams) but the energy consumed varied with the fat content. On the high-fat diet the women ate, on average, 2,700 kcal per day, compared with 2,090 kcal on the low-fat diet, and their weights changed accordingly.[1]

A similar experiment was conducted by James Stubbs at the UK Medical Research Council's Dunn Clinical Nutrition Centre in Cambridge, with Andrew Prentice, whose work on the energetics of obesity we met in Chapter 7. Six male volunteers spent three seven-day periods living in one of the institute's calorimeters so that their energy balance (intake–expenditure) could be measured. Each time, they were supplied with a different diet. They ordered food when they wanted, and were given dishes typically of 1 kg of food, from which they took as much as they desired and returned the rest. The results bore out those of Lissner's study. Energy balance was slightly negative (meaning a loss of weight if sustained in the longer term) on a low-fat, low-calorie diet, significantly positive (storing energy) on a high-fat, high-calorie diet. Again, the weight of food eaten each day, around 2 kg, was very similar between diets.[2] Very similar results were found in a US study based on individual days of feeding test meals that were more similar to typical American diets.[3]

These experiments show how adding fat can increase the calories in a given amount of food, and then, in turn, the number of calories that people will tend to eat. They feed into the concept called by nutritionists 'energy density'. This refers to the calorie content of a given weight of food. It is relevant because there is a lot of evidence that we get used to eating a certain weight of food at each meal. Let's just suppose that we are used to eating 1 kilogram per meal. If you refer back to 'Illustration of the difference between fats and carbohydrates as energy stores' on page 71, you will see immediately that 1 kilogram could mean a lot of calories, if it were rich in fat, for example, or not many if we were to eat mainly vegetables such as potatoes, with all the water they contain. To give some examples, for each 100 grams, raw celery comes in at 16 kcal, a typical breakfast cereal around 370 kcal, a pack of cookies I have in the cupboard (unopened, as it happens) 496 kcal, and a well-known confectionery bar 516 kcal. These differences in calories are determined mainly by the fat content (more fat = more calories) and the water content (the other way). You may remember that Mike Stroud fat-loaded the rations for his Antarctic crossing with Ranulph Fiennes, for exactly this reason.

The importance of this effect was brought home to me when a student in our laboratory, Katy Culling, persuaded volunteers to follow each of three different diets: one high in fat, one high in sugars and one high in complex carbohydrates (wholegrains, vegetables, starchy foods). The idea was to keep body weight constant, to examine the effects of the diets on blood lipids.[4] But when the volunteers were following the diet high in complex carbohydrates, they found it difficult to eat all the food they were prescribed. Their weight tended to drop, which (in this case) was not what we wanted. That's anecdotal, but other studies bear out the same message. In a cohort of over 2,000 breast-cancer survivors, there was a very strong relationship between dietary energy density and body weight,[5] and two meta-analyses have shown that higher habitual dietary energy density is associated with a greater tendency to gain weight.[6] These observations have prompted many people to suggest that those struggling with weight should be encouraged to eat a lower energy-density diet.[7] There are many scientific reports supporting this idea. In all fairness, though, I should say there is one in which the volunteers, followed for four years, did not show a loss of weight compared to controls.[8]

The major determinants of energy density, then, are the dietary fat content, and (working in the opposite direction) the water content. It's therefore not surprising that several studies have shown that a diet low in fat, hence with low energy density, leads to weight loss compared with a more typical 'Western' diet.[9] This does not go against the evidence I cited in the previous chapter, that those wishing to lose weight might do better on a low-carbohydrate diet: the main objective of the studies I've just listed was not weight loss. But it is all entirely in accord with what we know about those who have lost weight and then kept it off, as reviewed in the previous chapter: these people tend to follow a diet low in fat and to increase fruit and vegetable intake.

Apart from low fat content, a low-energy-density diet is typically characterised by plentiful fruit and vegetables. These contain a lot of water and are also fibre-rich, helping to bulk out meals (and keep the energy density low). A diet with low energy density might just be the key to being able to feel full at mealtimes, and yet keep body weight under control. But, you may say, fruits and vegetables are starchy, high-sugar foods. How can we reconcile that with the current popularity of low-carbohydrate diets? The answer is that we must distinguish better between different sorts of carbohydrate.

Sugar is sweet – but perhaps it's not helpful to your waistline

Sugars are carbohydrates. The current popularity of low-carbohydrate diets blurs the distinction between sugars and less-processed carbohydrate-rich foods. A meal rich in minimally processed fruit and vegetables (that is, raw or simply cooked), and low in fat, will have about as low an energy-density as any realistic meal can. But adding sugar into the diet is a sure way of *increasing* the energy density.

Of all the components of our diets, perhaps sugars lead to the most misunderstanding. In the UK we are advised to eat five portions of fruit and vegetables each day. But fruit contains sugar. Is that good or bad? Nutritionists draw a distinction between the sugars naturally present in fruit and vegetables, and sugars added to increase palatability. (Sugars present in juices extracted from fruit pose more of a dilemma, however, as I explain below.)

In 2015, three bodies independently presented guidelines for sugar consumption. In the UK, the Scientific Advisory Committee on Nutrition (SACN), which advises Government, published its report on 'Carbohydrates and Health'. SACN borrowed the term 'free sugars' from the World Health Organization, which issued guidelines on sugar consumption at the same time.[10] 'Free sugars' refers to all sugars added to foods, plus those naturally present in honey, syrups and un-sweetened fruit juices (although the definition of free sugars is more complex than might appear[11]). Sugars 'contained within the cellular structure of foods' are not included be-cause they are handled differently in our digestive systems.[12] (Milk sugar – lactose – is also excluded, mainly because of its lack of effect on dental caries. It adds calories, but at least it is usually accompanied by other beneficial nutrients such as protein and calcium.) The SACN report recommended that the population average intake of free sugars should not exceed 5 per cent of total dietary energy, a figure that they considered would help both energy balance and the problem of dental caries. The WHO report recommended that intake of free sugars should be reduced to below 10 per cent of total dietary energy, with a provisional recommendation to reduce it further to 5 per cent, mainly on the basis of evidence about dental caries. (These figures are not incompatible, as one refers to the population average, one to individuals.) At the same time, the US Government published the eighth edition of its *Dietary Guidelines for Americans, 2015–2020*.[13] They used the term 'added sugars' and recommended 'limiting calories from added sugars to no more than 10 per cent [of energy intake]'. Given that 'added sugars' will generally be less than 'free sugars', this is a less stringent recommendation than that in the UK or by the WHO.

I have heard strenuous discussion of the rights and wrongs of the definition of free sugars. A smoothie (a fruit purée) has more free sugars than the fruit from which it was prepared. But it is a very different thing to eat an apple than to drink a glass of apple juice pressed from it, or a smoothie made from it. The juice or the smoothie slip down easily, whereas the apple takes some chewing and fills one up with its bulk. A second glass of juice would also go down easily: a second apple might just seem too much. What's more, and this is a metabolic effect that we will look at again later, the speed with which sugars enter the bloodstream will be very different. Sugars trapped within the cellular structure of fruits and vegetables will be liberated, digested and absorbed more slowly than those already free in solution.

My very first PhD student, when I worked in Manchester, was Michael Goran. Michael worked with us on the effect of infections on energy metabolism. After that, he moved to the USA and worked with a number of obesity experts, making a name for himself through studies of obesity in young people, especially from the Hispanic areas of Los Angeles. He is now Professor of Pediatrics at the University of Southern California. Michael has come to believe firmly that sugar plays a very big role in obesity and metabolic problems starting in early life. He has recently published a book, *Sugarproof*, with Emily Ventura, giving practical advice on 'How to raise healthy kids in today's high sugar food environment, teach them to self-regulate sugar intake, and enjoy good food and good health for years to come'. Michael spent a year with us in Oxford around the time I retired from laboratory work and says that it was during this year that he began to formulate his ideas for *Sugarproof*. We had some interesting discussions. I remember saying to Michael that, of course, diet drinks such as diet cola are a great way of reducing sugar and calorie intake. Michael's response, completely to my surprise, was

'I wouldn't give that stuff to my kids. It's full of chemicals.' Since that time, evidence for the potentially harmful effects of the artificial sweeteners used in diet drinks has been increasing (although not necessarily at the levels that most of us are likely to consume). Furthermore, surprising though it might be, there is little or no evidence that these artificial sweeteners help to reduce calorie intake in the long term: they may encourage a 'sweet tooth'. The World Health Organization in 2023 released guidelines advising against the use of artificial sweeteners for weight control, and suggesting that we all need to get used to less sweet foods.[14]

Blaming sugar for various ills is not a new argument. *Pure, White and Deadly* was the catchy title of a book published by the British nutritionist John Yudkin, in 1972. (The subtitle was *How sugar is killing us and what we can do to stop it.*) It made the case that excess sugar consumption was responsible for many adverse outcomes, including obesity, type-2 diabetes and heart disease. These views were revolutionary at the time and led to criticism (especially from the sugar industry), but many people would now support them. More recently, other scientists have written on similar themes, including Robert Lustig with *Fat Chance: The Bitter Truth About Sugar* in 2012, and Gary Taubes, who has shared this adverse view of sugar in books, including *The Case Against Sugar* (2016), and an article in the *New York Times Magazine* in 2002 called 'What if it's All Been a Big Fat Lie?' One common theme here is a claim that reduction of fat in the diet has no benefits; indeed, that fat reduction may help fuel the obesity crisis. As I have explained, I don't believe that the evidence supports this; I think the opposite is true.

Veteran US obesity researcher George Bray has written about the potential role of high-fructose corn syrup in obesity. High-fructose corn syrup, known as isoglucose or glucose–fructose syrup in Europe, is a sweetener widely used in the food industry since its invention in the USA in the 1970s. It is made from cornstarch, which, like other starches, is a polymer of glucose. To make this into high-fructose corn syrup, the starch is hydrolysed (glucose units broken off) and an enzyme is used to convert some of the glucose to fructose, which is sweeter. Bray points out that, in the USA, consumption of high-fructose corn syrup increased ten-fold between 1970 and 1990. By 2004 it added on average 132 kcal per day to the American diet, and for high soft-drink consumers perhaps 316 kcal. The increase in high-fructose corn syrup consumption parallels closely the rise in American obesity.[15] That does not prove cause and effect, as many other things were changing over a similar period, but it does make high-fructose corn syrup a likely contributor to increasing body weight. In Europe and the USA the main sources of free sugars in the diet are 'sugar-sweetened beverages' (sodas or fizzy drinks), sweet foods (cakes, biscuits) and dairy desserts such as ice cream.[16]

A big question, not completely resolved in my view, is whether sugar in the diet is a bad thing simply because it contributes calories (calories that slip down easily: they don't need chewing or require slow digestion), or whether there are metabolic harms beyond the calorie content. Experts I have talked to have been equivocal about this. A common suggestion is that fructose is readily converted into fat for storage. Indeed, Robert Lustig says 'when you consume fructose, you're not consuming a carbohydrate, you're consuming fat'.[17] We have studied the short-term effects of fructose. There is no doubt that fructose increases the level of triacylglycerol (fat) in the bloodstream, although in our experiments the fatty acids in the blood were not formed directly from the fructose.[18] But so far as energy goes, although fructose is metabolised by a different pathway from glucose, it ends up as acetyl-CoA and will feed into the citric acid cycle along with all other nutrients. More generally, free sugars enter rapidly into the bloodstream and, in the case of glucose, will induce a rapid spike in insulin. Possibly, if that happens regularly, it will begin to down-regulate the sensitivity of the tissues to insulin, and potentially then increase the risk of type-2 diabetes. One measure of this is the glycaemic load (GL) of the diet – the product of the amount of carbohydrate, and its speed of raising glucose (the glycaemic index). And there is evidence that a habitual high-dietary glycaemic load is associated with an increased incidence of type-2 diabetes.[19]

I think a reasonable summary of the evidence is that added sugar is mainly of concern because it makes food tempting, but adds 'empty calories' (calories that bring no additional nutritional benefit); however, adverse metabolic events may follow when there is surplus energy intake. Luc Tappy in Lausanne has shown in a series of experiments that a high fructose intake causes deleterious metabolic effects, but that exercise will overcome these.[20] The clear message is that we should avoid sugars other than those within foods (such as fruit) so far as possible, and if we can't resist some, we need to exercise more to 'burn it off'.

Roughage takes centre stage

When I first met Theresa, now my wife of many years, and was introduced to her family, one topic of conversation at meal times seemed to be 'roughage'. This was new to me. My mother always cooked vegetables, but we never particularly thought about what they were doing for us – we just vaguely knew they were healthy. (Actually, I was commonly told that eating greens would make my hair curly: the last thing I wanted, since I already battled with frizzy locks.) Roughage referred to plant material that was not readily digested, and its supposed importance was that it helped to keep our bowel movements regular and soft, and hence led to a healthy bowel. It was not a topic much discussed in the medical literature until the Irish surgeon Denis Burkitt brought it to our attention in the early 1970s. Burkitt had spent much of his career in Africa, and was well known as the discoverer of the childhood cancer called 'Burkitt's lymphoma'. But he had also begun to take an interest in the very different patterns of disease in Africa and in Europe, and focused his attention on dietary fibre – the modern term for roughage. Burkitt reviewed many diseases of the gut that differ in occurrence between African and Western (developed) countries, such as appendicitis, haemorrhoids, diverticulitis and colon cancer. He suggested that the higher incidence in westernised countries was associated with a relative lack of fibre in the diet.[21] (I heard Burkitt speak about his work in the late 1970s. He encouraged all of us in the audience to examine our faeces and report to him the proportions of 'floaters' and 'sinkers', and whether we took a bran supplement.) The evidence for a protective role of dietary fibre against colon cancer has held up well over the years since.[22] Dietary fibre has other health benefits. A massive meta-analysis covering 135 million person-years of data showed strong protective effects of high-dietary fibre intake against cardiovascular disease, type-2 diabetes and, again, colon cancer.[23]

Our interest here, though, is in dietary fibre and energy balance. There is strong evidence from observational studies, as well as clinical trials, that high dietary fibre intake is associated with lower body weight, or less weight gain.[24] There may be several reasons for this.

One is simply that dietary fibre is 'filling'. It's difficult to overeat when your plate is full of fibre-rich foods. That is the concept of energy density that we looked at above.

Another effect of dietary fibre is that it interferes with our ability to digest nutrients. We saw in Chapter 2 that Wilbur

Atwater investigated the digestibility of carbohydrates, fats and proteins in different contexts, and found that diets high in vegetable matter, 'refuse' as he called it, reduced the digestibility of these nutrients by up to 10 per cent. That's potentially quite a lot of energy that goes down the pan, not into our bodies. There are more modern studies of this effect, involving volunteers eating diets or meals with varying amounts of added cereal fibre, and looking at faecal energy losses. Adding dietary fibre always results in increased faecal bulk, both water and solid matter, and indeed reduces the absorption of carbohydrates, fat and proteins, as Atwater found.[25] However, the effect depends on large amounts of dietary fibre, far greater than are consumed by most in the US or UK populations, and one study dismissed the addition of fibre as 'unlikely to induce a useful loss of calories in the management of obesity'.[26] It might not be the major reason to aim for a high fibre intake, but it could help. As we shall see shortly, some of the fibre will be broken down in the colon to produce metabolic products that include the gases hydrogen, methane and carbon dioxide. My friend Charles, an economist, hoped to pre-empt my writing of this book with his own contribution to weight management, *Fart Your Way to an Attractive Figure*. He was disappointed when I pointed him to recent data on human methane emissions, which are smaller in terms of calorie content than one might think from their wide reach.[27]

The effect of fibre on slowing down digestion is good for health. Fibre reduces the rate at which food leaves the stomach for the small intestine, and reduces the rate at which it is digested there. The rise in blood glucose after a meal, therefore, is slower when the meal is rich in fibre.[28] There are a number of systems in the body for sensing the arrival of nutrients – we looked very briefly at some of these in Chapter 5. They include receptors for nutrients, including glucose, within the circulation. This sensing contributes to knowing when we are full, and deciding when we want to eat next.[29] It seems entirely plausible that the longer the time that glucose is still entering the circulation after a meal, the longer will be our feeling that we don't need to eat again. Possibly related to this is a long-standing observation, but well documented, that obese people eat more quickly than the non-obese.[30] There could be many reasons for this, including the nature of the food eaten,[31] which affects eating rate, and to my knowledge there has not been a study showing that slowing the rate at which someone eats will reduce body weight. But still, it fits the idea that we should aim for a slower entry of nutrients into the circulation after a meal, which means eating plenty of fibre, and that in itself will reduce the speed of ingesting calories.

The role of the colon

What happens to the dietary fibre, which, by definition, cannot be digested in our stomach and small intestine, when it reaches the colon? This was not a major topic of scientific interest for many of the years that I studied nutrition and metabolism. The colon was considered as something akin to the garbage can: stuff collected there waiting to be disposed of. It has come to the forefront over the past couple of decades. And I accept that, because of that history, my view of the field may be a little more dismissive than it should be.

Anything that has not been digested in the small intestine arrives at the colon. This includes plant cell-wall components such as cellulose, which we cannot process with our own digestive enzymes. Some forms of starch that resist digestion also arrive here. Some starch forms crystals that block the action of the normal amylase digestive enzymes: this is called 'resistant starch'. In the colon, a vast colony of micro-organisms, mainly bacteria, gets to work in a process called fermentation. Estimates vary, but there are something like as many bacteria in the colon as we have human cells. These bacteria represent a vast diversity of species, some of which are generally considered 'beneficial', whereas others can be harmful.

These microorganisms salvage some energy that would otherwise be excreted in faeces. Some of the products of this fermentation are absorbed into the cells lining the colon. Among these is a group of fatty acids with two to four carbon atoms in their chains. These are called 'short-chain fatty acids' (SCFA), or sometimes 'volatile fatty acids', as they have low boiling points. This latter property also makes them 'smelly'. The most prominent are acetic acid (two carbons), propionic acid (three carbons) and butyric acid (four carbons). Butyric acid has a smell like milk that has gone off (a similar process). Denise Robertson, working as a post-doctoral researcher in my laboratory, studied the roles of these short-chain fatty acids in metabolism. She set up a method to measure them in blood samples. As Denise opened a bottle of butyric acid, and its vapour wafted across the lab, it instantly took me back to the long-forgotten smell of babies' nappies: full of fermented milk.

Acetic and propionic acids can be used in our tissues to make fatty acids or glucose. Butyric acid is used directly by the cells lining the colon, and appears to be beneficial in terms of reducing cancerous changes. Through the action of the colonic microorganisms, around 5–10 per cent of our energy intake can be salvaged. In herbivores, for example, cows or sheep, around 70 per cent of their energy requirement comes via the action of microorganisms in their intestinal tract. This, of course, is improving the overall efficiency of metabolism. We might, then, think that antibiotic use to kill some of the intestinal bacteria would result in lower energy harvesting and weight loss. But it is an old observation that animals treated with antibiotics tend to gain weight. Indeed, that is one reason why farm animals in many countries receive large doses of antibiotics: they act as growth promoters. (One suggestion is that they reduce competition between gut bacteria and the host animal for energy.[32]) Some studies in humans show that antibiotic use early in life predisposes to later obesity,[33] but we lack studies of whether there is an effect on obesity – and if so, in which direction – in adults.

The spectrum of microorganisms in the colon is referred to as the microbiome (like the genome or the metabolome). The relative proportions of the different species vary from person to person. It turns out that obese and lean people tend to have different bacterial species present. In particular, the ratio of two different families of bacteria, the Bacteroidetes and Firmicutes, differs. An early observation was that obese animals, such as the *ob/ob* mouse (described on page 92), have a 50 per cent reduction in the abundance of Bacteroidetes and an increased proportion of Firmicutes. This has been confirmed in most, but not all, studies in obese humans, and the ratio changes towards the 'lean' ratio when obese people diet to lose weight.[34] But is this cause or effect? Potentially, gut bacteria could influence appetite through signals released into the blood, or affect the ability of the body to harvest otherwise wasted energy.[35] In animals, faecal transplant experiments, in which faecal microorganisms from a lean animal (rats or mice have been used) are 'transplanted' into an obese animal, point to this being causal – that is, the type of microorganisms in the large intestine determines the body weight, rather than vice versa.[36] Human faecal transplantation is an established treatment for infection with the nasty bacterium *Clostridium difficile*. But, as yet, we do not have evidence of it being used successfully to alter body weight.

Whatever my reservations about the colonic microorganisms being the cause of obesity, I do think there is overwhelming evidence that keeping our colonic microorganisms happy is good for many aspects of health, including immunity. There are many supplements one can buy, supposedly to help achieve this. Prebiotics contain materials that are indigestible in the small intestine, and so feed the microorganisms in the colon. Probiotics contain live bacteria that are supposed to colonise directly (those that are not destroyed during the passage through the extreme acidity of the stomach). But, on the whole, a diet high in fibre-rich plant material will achieve many of the same benefits – and has other advantages, as we've just seen.

Your food is currently being (highly) processed

Some car enthusiasts will buy a kit of parts and spend time assembling their own vehicle. They will know exactly what is inside that car. But most of us let the manufacturer do it for us. And you can bet that no manufacturer is going to try to sell something that isn't ultra-sleek, attractive to look at, and full of labour-saving gadgets. And so it is with food. We are lucky in Oxford, where I live. There are several street markets where we can buy local fresh produce and take it home to create our own dishes. We don't eat most of it raw – we cook it or process it in other ways. Still, we know exactly what is in it. But for many people, this isn't the way of life. Fresh produce can be expensive. It's not always readily available. Working parents may struggle to find time to prepare meals from fresh ingredients. And the food manufacturers, just like the car makers, are ready to sell us things that they have devised – often in a laboratory – that will be tasty, almost irresistible, that might be advertised as 'low in sugar' or 'low in fat' but probably aren't low in calories, and that contain little fibre, but lots of things with chemical names. These are now generally called 'ultra-processed foods'. They have been described as 'inexpensive, [with] long shelf-life ... relatively safe from the microbiological perspective, provide important nutrients [that means mainly calories], and are highly convenient – often being either ready-to-eat or ready-to-heat'.[37] There are different definitions of ultra-processed foods. One widely used description is that this term refers 'to industrial formulations manufactured from substances derived from foods or synthesized from other organic sources. They typically contain little or no whole foods, are ready-to-consume or heat up, and are fatty, salty or sugary and depleted in dietary fibre, protein, various micronutrients and other bioactive compounds.'[38] The consumption of foods fitting these criteria increased rapidly in the early years of this century, with lower-middle-income countries showing the fastest growth in sales, although an international report in 2016 suggested that sales of these foods are levelling off.[39] A 2019 study showed that ultra-processed foods now contribute 57 per cent of our energy intake (on average) in the UK, and 65 per cent of our free sugars intake.[40] In Canada, ultra-processed foods accounted for 62 per cent of energy intake in a study from 2012, and it may well have increased since then.[41]

We have a lot of information on what consumption of these ultra-processed foods does to us. Some of it is anecdotal. Two British doctors, the late Michael Mosley and Chris van Tulleken, have independently described their own experiences eating such foods. Both describe how they felt lethargic, constipated and how they put on weight – but perhaps most strikingly, how they began to 'crave more junk food'.[42] But we also have scientific studies. US obesity researcher Kevin Hall, at the National Institutes of Health, studied twenty volunteers who lived for the duration of the experiment in the institute (so we can be sure about what they were eating). Half were offered a diet made up largely of ultra-processed foods, half a diet of largely unprocessed food; after two weeks, they switched and followed the other diet. They were provided with three meals per day and allowed to eat as much or as little as they desired. Crucially, the two diets were matched in proportions of carbohydrate, fat and protein and even in fibre and sugar content, and total calories offered (in this respect they were not typical ultra-processed foods). The results were very clear: volunteers offered the ultra-processed foods ate 500 kcal/day more, and gained weight, whereas on the un-processed diet they lost weight.[43] In the large-scale CARDIA study of over 3,000 people followed for fifteen years in the USA, eating 'fast-food' (largely ultra-processed) regularly was associated with weight gain.[44] And there's also information on the health effects of these foods. Many large studies in European and American populations show that higher con-sumption of ultra-processed foods is associated with increased risks of cardiovascular disease, type-2 diabetes, development of bowel cancers, and with higher mortality during up to fifteen years of follow-up.[45]

I did assume, in a rather prejudiced way, that some of the associations with ill-health might reflect the fact that those in lower-income brackets eat more ultra-processed food – and have, for multiple reasons, poorer health. But the data – lim-ited though they are – seem to prove me wrong. In the UK, those in lower economic groups tend to eat less minimally processed food, but not more ultra-processed than the more wealthy;[46] in a Canadian population, there was almost no dif-ference in ultra-processed food contribution to energy intake across income groups;[47] and in Brazil, it was the better-off who consumed more ultra-processed foods than those less well off.[48]

As I write this, there is discussion about whether specific components of ultra-processed foods – for example, emulsi-fiers[49] – lead to ill health, or whether it's more simply the fact that these are generally high-calorie, low-fibre foods. From our point of view, that's what matters. Cakes and biscuits baked at home, which may not count as ultra-processed, are still high-calorie and low-fibre and not helpful to your calorie balance![50]

Many writers on 'healthy living' share the view that we should try to eat mainly, or even exclusively, minimally processed food. Rangan Chatterjee, another British doctor who writes about healthy lifestyles, advises in *Feel Great, Lose Weight*: 'eat more real food', defining that as 'food that's minimally processed, close to its natural state and instantly recognizable', and suggests 'basing your meals around wholefoods'. This is essentially saying avoid ultra-processed foods. It's a common theme now – and, of course, it fits exactly with what we discussed above about energy density. But it would be a mistake to use this food classification blindly. A survey by the British Nutrition Foundation (BNF) found that most British adults were, anyway, unaware of the terminology.

> When given a list of foods and asked which they would classify as ultra-processed, just 8 per cent selected canned baked beans, 9 per cent low-fat fruit yogurt, 12 per cent ice cream, 19 per cent prepackaged sliced bread from a supermarket, and 28 per cent breakfast cereals with added sugar, despite all of the above being classed ... as ultra-processed.[51]

In striving to introduce some balance to the discussion, the BNF points out that 'many foods are inedible without some form of processing ... Home cooking is also a form of processing, and techniques such as boiling, fermenting and salting have been used for thousands of years.'[52] The idea that we should view beans on toast as unhealthy has been described as 'half-baked'.[53] We need a balanced view, and we all need to learn to read nutritional labelling, which is the only way, in the end, to know just what you are eating. (See Appendix, page 253, for more information on nutrition labelling.)

Calorie labelling

This book is about calories – calories taken in, calories expended – so of course I must be in favour of calorie counting and calorie labelling, mustn't I? The answer, I am afraid, is 'yes' and 'no'.

Yes, I do think that it's useful to have some idea of what we are taking in. In 2022 the UK Government introduced mandatory calorie labelling of menus in larger catering establishments, following the lead of the USA in 2018. It has been very controversial. Some argued against it on the basis that we should not be 'nannied' by the Government. Others argued that a single figure for calories does not impart much information – the impact on body weight depends also on nutrient content. But I think it has to be helpful to have an idea of what one is eating; then one can make choices. Nobody would argue against labelling potential antigens in foods because it represents a 'nanny state'. But I do understand an objection from those who argue that calorie labelling may have adverse effects for those with eating disorders.

Why, then, do I say that I am not necessarily in favour? The reason is that calorie labelling, for all its apparent scientific basis, going back to the work of Atwater, is an imprecise science. We saw that Atwater rounded off his figures for the calorie yield of nutrients. He knew that the actual caloric value depended upon the composition of the food eaten. Cambridge obesity scientist Giles Yeo addresses these issues in his book *Why Calories Don't Count*. As Yeo says, we eat food, not calories. And he goes on to suggest better calorie values. I am a great believer in collating data on a spreadsheet: my own medical history, the output from our solar panels, my bank account: all on spreadsheets. But I wouldn't bother with a spreadsheet for calories. I don't think it would be particularly helpful, because of the imprecision of the values. And, of course, I would really struggle to add 'calories out' to my spreadsheet. That would be largely guesswork.

But – when I look at the menu in our local branch of a well-known coffee chain, and I see that that oh-so-tempting White Chocolate Mocha Frappuccino Blended Beverage will provide me with 251 kcal (about one-tenth of my daily energy), whereas I could have a filter coffee for 24 kcal (a little more if I add milk), surely that's useful information to guide my choice? Or, at a pizza chain restaurant in Oxford, if I can choose between the Margherita at 807 kcal or the rectangular Calabrese at 1,275 kcal, I don't see how that can fail to be helpful. These values are sufficiently different that, even with the imprecision that I have mentioned, I know that there will be a substantial difference in calories between the extremes. (Some anecdotal evidence suggests that a diner seeing a high-calorie cake, for example, might decide to share with a friend.[54])

There's a limited amount of scientific evidence on the effect of calorie labelling on consumption. It's a difficult topic to study, and relatively new. In a 2018 review of the evidence available, the authors felt that there was some evidence that calorie labelling reduced calorie consumption, but that the research was not conclusive.[55] There is also evidence from the USA that calorie labelling may drive down the calorie content of new items added to the menu.[56]

I also think that nutritional labelling is important. Here's an example. I see that breakfast cereals are now classified as ultra-processed food, which disappoints me, as I enjoy a good bowl of cereal to start my day. (I won't change that. Some are more processed than others. Some have more added sugar or fat. The British Heart Foundation gives you suggestions as to which are healthier choices.[57]) But how about granolas? I'm looking at a recipe online for making what will, apparently, be 'the very best granola'. It includes oil, either coconut or olive, which 'helps make this granola crisp and irresistible', and it is 'naturally sweetened' with maple syrup or honey rather than refined sugar, which may indeed improve the taste but adds the same calories. A quick glance at the nutritional labelling of supermarket granolas will tell you that they provide well over 400 kcal per 100 grams. One brand I like produces a honey granola at 474 kcal per 100 grams. But the same brand's fruity muesli comes in at 349 kcal per 100 grams. (That's a very clear example of the effect of added fat on energy density.) Given that I eat this every day, my choice is clear to me. And I don't think I lose any pleasure by choosing one over the other – perhaps I have unconsciously, over the years, taken to preferring things that I feel are healthier. When I am looking for a new brand of cereal, I will look at the nutritional labelling for calories, fat, sugars and salt (I want all these to be low) and fibre (which I want to be high), all of which can differ considerably: compare a few brands and you'll see the differences.

Alcohol

One more topic we need to discuss when considering calories is alcohol. A nice cool, clear glass of wine – what could be more innocent-looking? But alcohol is processed metabolically through the same pathways as all other nutrients, and feeds acetyl-CoA (discussed in Chapter 4) into the citric acid cycle for oxidation. In fact, as the body has no means to store alcohol or its breakdown products, it's oxidised as quickly as it's broken down, driving other nutrients into storage. My research group did some work on alcohol at one time. I was interested in the question: if, indeed, alcohol is providing calories, then in some way it must feed information to our fat stores to increase their energy storage. How is that transmitted? We didn't really answer that question, but we had some interesting experiences along the way. Gin was provided for our research by a local off-licence. We discovered that the students who were involved in the project had a much greater tolerance to large quantities of gin than did the senior members of the group (myself particularly). The research was sparked off by a suggestion that there is a pathway for metabolising alcohol that simply wastes the energy. That would have been good news for drinkers. But now it seems that this only occurs in those whose livers have been badly damaged by long-term excessive drinking. The Atwater system gives alcohol an energy value of 7 kcal per gram. A typical drink in the pub (glass of wine, pint of beer) will provide 150–200 kcal. And, of course, with a nice drink beside you, it may be more tempting to have something to eat to go with it – and perhaps another drink to follow up. It's all obvious but potentially overlooked. Low-to-moderate alcohol consumption is not consistently associated with obesity, but heavy drinking is.[58] There may be many lifestyle factors that complicate the relationship in moderate drinkers.

Evidence-based eating – a summary

What have we learned from all the above? Losing weight is not easy – keeping it off might be even harder. It requires a change in lifestyle. However you lose weight, you will probably need to look for a different lifestyle to keep it off. Here's my distillation of the evidence for eating in a way that minimises your chances of weight gain.

First, eliminate so far as possible added and free sugars. But that definitely does not mean avoiding fruit which, in normal amounts, has many health benefits and adds fibre to the diet. Unfortunately, the evidence does not support the idea that taking diet drinks instead will help the situation, so perhaps develop a taste for water (sparkling water can add a little something), or unsweetened tea (including the wide range of herbal teas) or coffee. Also look at nutrition labelling with an eye on sugars: some cereals, for example, have more than others. Do the same for fat. I was going to write 'eliminate unnecessary fats', but actually not much fat is in any sense necessary. Be wary of claims about 'healthy fats': they all add calories. Yes, we do need to take in small amounts of certain polyunsaturated fatty acids that we cannot make for ourselves, but in tiny amounts. Probably the n-3 (omega-3) fatty acids in fish are good for us, but the evidence is not consistent on this – and they still add calories. Increase fibre intake as much as possible: most of us eat far less fibre than the recommended 30 grams per day. All these changes will reduce the energy density of the diet and make it easier to reduce 'calories in' without feeling too deprived of food. And check package labelling for anything that might be overly processed: what you are looking out for are high calories, fat, sugars and salt[*] and low fibre (usually expressed per 100 grams).

Furthermore, physical activity has to become part of daily life. Becoming more physically active will bring many health benefits as well as aiding weight control. It will help because physical activity uses calories, but also quite probably because it changes our mindset and our relationship to food. At the very least, make sure you break up sedentary time with regular walks around the house or office.

Translating that into foods, fruit juices and sodas (fizzy

---

[*] High salt content is a concern for many people because it may raise blood pressure; nothing to do with calories.

drinks) must become occasional treats. Honey and preserves should be used in moderation. Regard all sweet things with a sceptical eye. Frying should be for rare occasions. To take an example, 220 grams of boiled potatoes (a typical portion) will provide around 170 kcal, with 0.2 grams of fat, whereas the same amount of chips (fries in the USA) will give you 690 kcal with 32 grams of fat – four times the energy density.[59] Think about reducing spreads on bread, and consider changing to skimmed milk, which gives you most of the nutritional benefits of whole or semi-skimmed milk but less fat and fewer calories. (You get used to it after a while.) Do everything you can to increase fibre intake in the form of fruit, vegetables and wholegrain foods. Of course, alcohol intake should be limited – remembering that alcohol provides calories that may even encourage you to eat and drink more. Most nutritionists – and the UK and US governments[60] – would also add: consume one or two portions of fish (one of which should be oily) each week, but this is about health, not body weight. Calorie labelling of food or drink consumed away from home should be seen as a useful guide: there will be big variations between drinks or dishes, and often a lower-calorie option will be just as tasty, or a high-calorie choice, if very tempting, might be ideal to share with a friend.

None of the above rules out treats or lazy days. We need to keep an eye on our regular diet, without becoming obsessive. And choosing lower-calorie foods will often mean choosing foods that are good for our health in other ways. The beauty of believing that 'a calorie is a calorie', so far as body weight goes, is that there are no foods you *cannot* eat: you just need to consider the calorie content, and some things should be occasional treats rather than a feature of everyday eating. The story of energy balance has shown that we must think in the long term. Trends matter, day-to-day fluctuations much less. That's one reason, I think, why regular weighing has been shown to help weight control: you can see trends emerging above the noise of days that vary in what we eat and what we do, and when weight fluctuations reflect body water more than body fat.

Of course, none of that will be a surprise, but I reiterate it because I hope to have convinced you that these recommendations are more than 'This is what I think you should do – based on my own experiences'. They all come firmly from the scientific evidence.

Eating for health, eating for body weight

In Chapter 1, I distinguished what we might think of as a 'healthy diet' – one that reduces disease – from one that is good for body weight. They are not necessarily the same. If we now come back to the last section of Chapter 1, we will see that, as I rather promised there, there's very little difference between what the science tells us we should eat to control our body weight, and what we should eat for more general health. That's no surprise really, given that body weight and metabolic health are so closely related. But, you may well say, we probably, deep down, all know that. So, how come we are where we are today? My answer to that is to point out how much things have changed to make it more and more difficult to eat in this healthy way.

12

Calories in–calories out: The delicate balance

We have come full circle. I said at the beginning that my belief is that our weight trajectory is based on the well-understood principle of 'calories in–calories out'. I've shown you how this idea developed over several centuries, and pointed out the many difficulties that people have in accepting it, not least because of our natural tendency to judge someone's eating behaviour (and, indeed, metabolism) from snapshot observations; and how scientists have for too long failed to appreciate the difficulty of capturing that information in an objective way.

But, to return to the argument made by those opposing this view: how come, then, that decades of public-health advice to eat less and exercise more have failed to dent the increase in overweight and obesity in many countries? This argument seems so powerful that it has convinced many that we don't correctly understand the forces that shape our body weight. My view, shared, I am pleased to say, by at least a few other experts, is that our ability to regulate in any way our body weights has been overwhelmed by changes in our environment: changes that tempt us to eat more, and to be less active. Yes, the human body has mechanisms that should help to keep body weight stable within reasonable limits, but these mechanisms evolved more to protect us in times of food shortage than to help us manage when food is plentiful.

I imagine Antoine Lavoisier looking out at today's world. In his time, the focus of his work was to increase agricultural production so that everyone might have sufficient food. Or even Wilbur Atwater, who, just over 100 years ago, would have had similar concerns about increasing the food supply. What, then, has changed so much in the past few decades, even since I started work in this field in the 1970s? In that time, worldwide obesity has nearly tripled.[1]

Firstly, not our genes. Yes, we have continued to evolve as I explained in Chapter 10, but not over that short period. As I've discussed earlier, our genes help to explain where in the distribution of human body weights we lie, but not where the average of this distribution is located: that is dependent upon our environment, and that is what has changed.

I am afraid that I discount government data on energy intake. As I outlined in Chapter 1, data in the UK and the USA seem to show that adult energy intake has, if anything, decreased over this period while physical activity may have increased. But all these data are based on self-reporting. We have seen just how misleading that may be. My guess is that one effect of the decades of advice to eat less and exercise more is that self-reported behaviours will change in exactly that way, while actual behaviours may well not have done.

We have seen many so-called advances in food technology. High-fructose corn syrup was introduced into our food supply around 1970.[2] Ultra-processed foods have come along since then. As emphasis has shifted from low-fat to low-sugar, we have seen new products aimed at meeting each of these, but they are not necessarily low in calories.

There has been a big increase in eating out. Since the UK's Office for National Statistics first started tracking the contribution made by different sectors to the UK economy in 1992, the value of spending on eating out has doubled. Over the same period, the amount spent on food and drink for consumption at home has risen just 50 per cent.[3] In the USA, the amount spent on eating and drinking out has gone from $200 billion in 1992 to nearly $900 billion in 2021.[4] And a lot of that eating out is likely to involve fast foods, consumption of which, as we have seen, is associated with a tendency to put on weight. What's more, there has been a well-documented increase in portion sizes since the 1970s, still ongoing, in parallel with the rise in obesity.[5] I am not saying that there's anything wrong with eating out, but it does mean that one loses control over what goes into a meal and how much of it we might eat. In the restaurants in our locality, it is much easier to find burgers, kebabs and pizzas than it is to find a dish that I would reckon to be very high in vegetable, and hence, fibre content.

As I write this, I have just returned from the USA where half our family lives (so I do experience life in both the USA and the UK). We went out to a diner for brunch. I was impressed to see, at either end of the table, large bottles of what I took to be maple syrup. (Impressed only because I was thinking how many sugar maple trees there must be in the USA.) In fact, they were pure fabrications – made of corn syrup, high-fructose corn syrup and various chemicals. This tempting stuff provides no nutritional value – no protein, fibre, vitamins or useful minerals, for example. But it's so easily added to the large plates of pancakes or 'French toast' that we all ordered. I am pretty sure that wasn't available to earlier generations.

We are also losing the ability to cook for ourselves. Too many families have given up home cooking with fresh vegetables as my grandmother and my mother would have done. An experiment by the UK food writer and broadcaster Hugh Fearnley-Whittingstall in the BBC programme *Britain's Fat Fight* involved offering free fruit and vegetables from a barrow in a poor area of northern England. While people were happy to take an apple or an orange, they were reluctant to take a cauliflower or a cabbage, let alone a celeriac, because they simply didn't know what to do with it. Education in cooking and nutrition has almost disappeared. The UK Government supposedly reintroduced cookery lessons in England's secondary schools for children aged eleven to fourteen.[6] Education on food preparation and healthy eating is part of the National Curriculum in all parts of the UK. I conducted a poll of my five grandchildren, then aged eleven to sixteen, who live each side of the Atlantic. They were receiving little or nothing, other than L, aged eleven, in the USA who has two weeks each winter on health topics, and A, aged sixteen, in the UK who says, 'Did it for a few months in Year 8 [ages twelve to thirteen].' (Fortunately, my grandchildren all learned to cook from their excellent parents, but not all youngsters will be so lucky.)

Linked to that is the idea that 'healthy eating is too expensive'. In the UK, a 2022 report by the Food Foundation claimed that 'Healthy nutritious food is nearly three times more expensive than obesogenic unhealthy products.'[7] Our World in Data claim that 'A healthy, nutritious diet is much more expensive than a calorie sufficient one. As a result, three billion people cannot afford a healthy diet.'[8] There is experimentation on both sides of the Atlantic in changing this by offering healthy foods as medical prescriptions. Several programmes in the USA were evaluated by researchers at Tufts University, Boston and the University of Massachusetts at Worcester, MA. These programmes, in which participants were offered vouchers or credit cards to spend on healthy foods at farmers' markets and grocery stores with a median value of $63 (£50) per month, increased intake of fruit and vegetables, and led to improvements in glucose control and blood pressure and a fall in weight: and, importantly in the present context, an increase in food security (the ability to buy food).[9]

On the 'calories out' side, we have seen so many changes that reduce our ability, or our desire, to increase physical activity. In all fairness, though, I must mention here recent data from an international consortium of researchers who have combined their data on people's total energy expenditure measured with doubly labelled water. These show that, in Europe and the USA, total energy expenditure has declined steadily since the late 1980s, as we might expect; but simultaneous measurements of *resting* energy expenditure seem to show that this is the component that has declined, not activity-related expenditure.[10] These data are puzzling and go against what we seem to observe in our everyday lives. It's not the place here to discuss how they could be misleading, but I would note that as a general principle in science, it's accepted that when new results challenge what we have previously believed, this calls for more experimentation to confirm the new thinking.

The facts suggest a different picture. Adults in Britain think that they watch an average of less than twenty hours of television a week, or around three hours a day, but official statistics collected by the Broadcasters' Audience Research Board (BARB) show that the true average in 2010 was more than thirty hours a week, or over four hours a day. The amount we watch is increasing: the BARB average for all ages (including children) is twenty-eight hours a week, which is three hours more than in 2001, not including the television we now watch on equipment other than our TV sets.[11] Figures are similar in the USA but show a recent downward trend, presumably as more people switch to other types of screen for entertainment and information.[12] (In the National Weight Control Registry database, hours of television viewing is strongly related to weight regain.[13]) And, of course, the time we spend looking at all screens is increasing – something that may have adverse consequences not just for our body weight, but also (in children especially) for our eyesight.[14]

Our travel patterns have changed. Car ownership has increased greatly in the UK: the proportion of households with a car rose from 52 to 78 per cent over the fifty years from 1971; over the same period, the number of households with two or more vehicles rose from 8 to 33 per cent.[15] In the USA, car ownership has always been higher, with 60 per cent of families owning a car in 1929;[16] in 2021 only 8 per cent of households did not have a car, and 22 per cent had three or more.[17] In 1963 the UK Government launched the Buchanan Report on Traffic in Towns. Although this was a well-meaning attempt to show how towns could be replanned to cope with the rise in motor car ownership, it has been blamed by many for urban blight, making roads unfriendly to pedestrians and cyclists, and destroying some town centres.[18] There is no doubt that children are much less likely to play outside than those who grew up in the immediate post-war years (such as myself).[19]

The possible good news is that, at least in Europe, things may be changing in the right direction. Successive governments and local authorities have sought to promote active travel (walking and cycling), and the trends are generally level or increasing. But still, in 2020, 66 per cent of adults in England agreed that 'it is too dangerous for me to cycle on the roads',[20] and a recent wave of introductions of low-traffic neighbourhoods, designed to make residential roads more attractive for walking, cycling and recreation has met very vocal opposition (and, as I write this, is being reconsidered by the government). Active travel in the USA remains lower than in many European countries: a 2011 comparison showed that the proportion of all trips made by walking in Germany was about 2.5 times that in the USA; for cycling, the difference was nearer ten-fold, and public transport use was also much higher in Germany.[21] And, everywhere we go, we find energy-saving devices: more escalators in larger shops, for example, travelators in airports, electric bikes and scooters for hire in cities.

None of those things changing over the same period as the increase in obesity proves cause and effect. I've pointed that out before, in connection with high-fructose corn syrup for example. But I think the mass of these changes in our environment, all going the same way, is sufficiently convincing that I don't see a need for alternatives to the 'calories in–calories out' model. Our innate regulatory mechanisms are overwhelmed. Not everyone's, of course. Yes, 64 per cent of the UK population (2019 data), 75 per cent of the US population are overweight or obese,[22] but let's not forget that means that 25–35 per cent are not. And that accords with just what we know about the genetics that underlie our body weight. As I mentioned earlier in this chapter, our genes haven't changed: but the environment has altered in such a way as to move the centre point of our weight distribution firmly towards the heavier side.

What, then, can we do? I feel it only right, having written and expected you to read eleven chapters of science, to say how I think things must change if we want to make it easier for everyone to balance their calories in and out.

At the individual level, I accept that there's no point in reiterating 'eat less and exercise more'. But there are things we have learned, by looking at the evidence, that may help us to change the way we live to achieve those ends. It's not an original thought that we need to return to eating less processed food, but the evidence on this is absolutely clear. Meals have to be based so far as possible on relatively unprocessed vegetables. Plenty of fruit and vegetables both help us to feel fuller and benefit our health in many ways. (There's a separate argument, that vegetable-based diets are better for the environment that I won't get into here, although I am not denying its importance.) I think it's no coincidence that, while I have been concentrating on energy balance, there have been many studies on eating for health, especially cardiovascular health. And universally those studies show that diets rich in fruit, vegetables, wholegrains and fibre, and low in processed meat and high-fat foods, are the healthiest[23] – interestingly, something my grandparents might have told me, but that I can now confirm based on many years of scientific evidence.

It's not up to me to tell you how to include physical activity in your daily lives. But what we have learned is that anything you can do is useful, provided that it doesn't lead you to compensate by eating more. Jim Hill, a US obesity expert involved with the National Weight Control Registry, tells me that most of those who have kept weight off manage the exercise side by walking. Remember that all physical activity is good for health, and that sedentary behaviour – sitting at your computer or in front of the television – is bad for health, and for energy balance. Breaking up sedentary times with movement (this might count as NEAT, see page 120) has to become the norm, and more businesses should provide facilities to do this, perhaps including modern so-called sit-and-stand desks.

I am not suggesting that we all lead the life of a monk or nun. Yes, we need to change what we eat but we don't need to starve ourselves and be miserable: we can still for the most part feel satisfied after a meal, although we might restrict some items to occasional treats. And we don't need to start pulling sledges across a wilderness or even go out and jog regularly (although I would advocate that if you can). Just incorporating more movement into your daily life may be enough to get your calories into balance. But, in the end, I am not naive, I know that everyone knows all that – although not, perhaps, the strength of the evidence behind it. And still we struggle: some more than others, largely, we know, because of our genetics. What, then, is the answer?

Some believe that the answer will come from drugs that help us to regulate our body weight. I am not alone in thinking that this cannot be the way the world moves forward. As one popular medical website puts it, 'drugs won't cure obesity. And that's OK, because obesity isn't a disease to be cured.'[24] *Times* journalist Alice Thomson puts it like this: 'So there we have it. Big food companies have been fattening us up for 50 years but big pharma will save us. Both industries are making vast profits ...'[25]

Instead, we need governments to change their attitudes on many levels. We know that this can be effective. In Japan, companies have since 2008 been required by law to measure their employees' waist circumference (a measure of abdominal obesity) every year. This is part of a healthy culture which includes, for example, some companies offering Amazon gift cards to those who take at least 8,000 steps a day. Education starts at school, where teachers eat with their pupils and explain the importance of a healthy diet. Absence from work through sickness is much less than in the UK, and obesity in Japan is unusual – rates are the lowest in the developed world.[26] In the 1970s, the governor of the Finnish province of North Karelia decided something had to be done about the very high prevalence of heart disease in the region – men were dropping dead in their forties and fifties. The diet was largely based on locally reared fatty pork with few vegetables. Over the next thirty years, a number of programmes aimed at healthier eating, more active lifestyles and smoking cessation improved the inhabitants' health enormously, with an 80 per cent reduction in heart disease in men.[27] That programme was aimed at reducing heart disease rather than weight loss. Obesity was relatively uncommon in the region.[28] But it shows how effective top-down intervention might be.

In contrast, a 2021 report on the government's approach to obesity in England identified '14 government strategies published from 1992 to 2020 containing 689 wide-ranging policies. Policies were largely proposed in a way that would be unlikely to lead to implementation; ... the majority ... relied on individuals to make behaviour changes rather than shaping external influences ...'[29] Another report found that 'None of the strategies developed over the last three decades has set out a credible long-term goal for what the government wants to achieve, backed up by evidence-based policies. No departments currently prioritise obesity ...'[30] International experience with 'sugar taxes' has been positive, but governments are generally unwilling to take this further with levies on other unhealthy foods, or even, in the UK at present, banning 'two-for-one' deals on unhealthy food.

But we need more than what UK obesity psychologist John Blundell calls 'tinkering with aspects of the food supply'. He goes on to ask: 'Can this happen in a capitalist system in which key commodities (especially food and transport) are driven by the need to maintain economic growth? Such a system ... controls people's behaviour to the same extent as an overtly authoritarian regime.'[31] It would be sad to end on the note that capitalism and obesity must inevitably go hand-in-hand. I would argue, though, that just as capitalism has to reinvent itself to adapt to the current environmental crisis, so it must in order to deal with our health. And there are undoubted opportunities, of which the sudden increase in sales of bicycles during the Covid-19 pandemic is but one example.[32]

Finally, I have throughout tried not to make this a personal account. I am a scientist and I wanted to write a science-based book. But I have hinted in several places that I am one of the lucky ones who does not particularly have a 'weight problem'. I thought it only fair, then, to say something about the lifestyle that I largely share with my wife, Theresa. In fact, I did begin to gain weight in a way I wasn't happy with in my thirties, as many people do. I had started the difficult work on metabolism in trauma patients in Manchester that occupied me for ten years. We had two growing children and weren't particularly well off. We shopped locally as cheaply as we could, including cheaper fatty cuts of meat or burgers, and we bought large tubs of margarine. The empty margarine tubs made great storage containers, so we piled them up in the kitchen. One day I looked at this pile and thought *Oh dear, where has all that fat gone?* (I was well enough advanced as a metabolic scientist to know the answer.) We fairly quickly gave up spreading fat on bread, and cut down on other dietary fat considerably. At the same time, I collected my rusty bicycle, unused since student days, from my parents' house and started cycling to work. Gradually my weight dropped to a level I was happy with. Of course, this experience just reinforced my growing belief in the doctrine of 'calories in–calories out'.

In more recent years, many people have asked me, when I give a lecture, 'Do you have some professional secret?' And, although I always deny it, perhaps I do in a way, having studied the science of energy balance for so many years. As I wrote in earlier chapters, I was struck by the description of those who have successfully managed to maintain weight loss, those in the National Weight Control Registry particularly. *Oh*, I thought many times, *that's just what we do*. We both enjoy our food and look forward to meals, but our diet is generally low in fat and high in vegetables and fruit, similar to that described by those in the Registry. For many reasons I won't go into here, we don't eat meat and so we avoid the fat in cheaper meat cuts or products such as burgers. (However, we both eat what others might consider large amounts of cheese, because we like it and because it is such a good source of animal protein and calcium, we accept the calories.) I think we are restrained over sweet things. We usually have cake and biscuits in the house, but they last a long time. We do quite often use a phrase coined by my mother, Enid: 'It's not worth the calories.'

I think equally importantly, though, we both do what we can to be physically active. And I do realise that's not so easy for everyone. I am lucky to have been able to keep jogging all my life, and, since that decision I made in my thirties, to have been able to cycle to work for much of my career. (That has determined our choices of where to live.) We walk or cycle locally and use our car only when there's no alternative. And when travelling we always walk up and down escalators, take the stairs when it's reasonable, and walk beside the travelators in airports – it has just become a habit to do this, part of our way of life. I get frustrated when we find ourselves trapped behind young people standing still on a down-escalator. Our holidays almost always involve something physical (mainly walking) – we prefer mountains to beaches or cruise ships. Also, we both weigh ourselves regularly and might make some adjustments when needed – another feature we have in common with successful weight-losers.

How much of this way of life is down to our genetics? I can't say. To me, of course, especially when I head out for an early winter's morning run, it can feel as though I am being 'sensible and strong willed'! But, again, as a scientist, I know a lot of that must come from our genes – I can't take credit for it. Also, I acknowledge that we are well-educated, we understand what we need to do, and we live in a relatively affluent part of a city where there are many people living similar lifestyles and there is good public transport. But, still, I do think that there are aspects of this lifestyle that would not be too difficult for many people who have a weight problem to adopt.

Here, then, is the long and the short of it. Our environment has changed dramatically over the past few decades. Some of us are lucky to be able to cope with this, perhaps because of lucky genes, partly because we live in the right circumstances. There are, though, things that shine out from the large body of research on energy balance that can guide us all as to how to resist these malign influences: changing the way we eat, without necessarily having to be hungry, and especially doing all we can to keep physically active.

Clearly, however, many will still struggle against this tide of influences leading them to exercise less and eat more calories than their parents' generation might have done. Then only government action can solve this. And most governments have signally failed to act in the way that's needed. Their excuses are to do with not wanting to interfere with personal choice (the 'nanny state'), not wanting to tell businesses what to do or increase their taxes, or make food more expensive for families who struggle anyway financially. At a local level, our transport authority (Oxfordshire County Council) has started an initiative to make streets more attractive for people walking and cycling, but this has not been entirely successful (motor traffic is displaced elsewhere) and has met enormous and very vocal opposition, as has also happened in other parts of the country. And yet a recent study shows that, in the UK, if everyone were a healthy weight, the NHS would save nearly £14bn annually,[33] so there should be a financial incentive for governments to act.

I end by reiterating what many of you will have recognised from the beginning: there are no tricks. Our body-weight trajectory is determined by the balance between calories in, and calories out. Each side of this equation can be altered to make it balance. This can come from our personal choices, but these need reinforcement through education, and through government policies on food supply and on transport. Arguments against this energy balance model are simply distracting us from what must be done.

Appendix

Nutrition labelling

Since I have several times advised you, the reader, to look at the nutrition labelling on products that you might eat, it may be useful to provide a little more information about what you are looking at.

In the UK, food-product labelling is (at the time of writing) aligned with that in the European Union (EU).[1] US Food and Drug Administration Regulations are broadly similar, although they are based on typical portion sizes (which, the regulations acknowledge, have increased in recent years).[2] The explanations below are based on UK/EU labelling.

This Appendix won't cover health claims. In the EU at present only two health claims relating to body weight are approved. One covers meal replacements ('soup and shake diets' as described in Chapter 10). The other covers glucomannan, a type of dietary fibre. Before you rush out to buy this, note that probably any type of fibre would help in the same way, and the effect on body weight is pretty minimal.[3]

Back-of-pack labelling

Most packaged foods must have nutrition labelling on the back of the pack, in a standardised format. This is expressed for a given weight (100 grams), or volume (100 millilitres) for liquids, and may also be given per typical portion. Required information is energy, fat and saturated fat content (saturated being part of total fat), carbohydrate and sugar content (sugar being part of total carbohydrate), protein content and salt content. Information on fibre, vitamins and minerals and other components (such as unsaturated fats) is optional.

In practice, most manufacturers include fibre. Here is some typical labelling, from two well-known brands of cereal, with explanation. (I found the explanation by putting lots of labelling into a spreadsheet so that I could see what the manufacturers are doing.)

Breakfast cereal 1

Component	Value, per 100 grams	Explanation	Value, per typical serving (37.5 grams)
Energy, kilojoules (kJ)	1531	Value in kJ is value in kcal × 4.2	574
Energy, kcal	362	This is not, as I once thought, the energy value when combusted. It's calculated as explained just below the table and represents metabolisable energy rather than total energy.	136
Fat, grams	2.0	In this case, there is no added fat; this will be naturally present in the grains from which it is mostly made.	0.8
– of which, saturates	0.6		0.2
Carbohydrate, grams	69	This does not include fibre, although that is mostly a form of carbohydrate. This is 'metabolisable' carbohydrate.	26
– of which, sugars	4.2	This cereal has added sugar.	1.6
Fibre, grams	10		3.8
Protein, grams	12		4.5
Salt, grams	0.3	Not relevant to body weight, but important for people with a tendency to high blood pressure.	0.1

Energy here in kcal is calculated as: (carbohydrate × 4) + (fat × 9) + (protein × 4) + (fibre × 2): in other words, using the Atwater factors that we looked at in Chapter 2.

How should we interpret these numbers – what are we looking for? This is easiest to see by comparing it to an apparently similar product:

Breakfast cereal 2

Component	Value, per 100 grams Cereal 1	Value, per 100 grams Cereal 2	Comments
Energy, kilojoules (kJ)	1531	1852	Marked difference (rather less for a typical portion of say, 40 grams).
Energy, kcal	362	441	
Fat, grams	2.0	14.8	And that's why! Added fat in cereal 2.
– of which, saturates	0.6	2.8	And, of course, more saturated fat, although both are high as a percentage of total fat.
Carbohydrate, grams	69	64	Seems similar – but look at Sugars, below.
– of which, sugars	4.2	13.5	More sugars in Cereal 2, so Cereal 1 is preferable in that respect.
Fibre, grams	10	6.2	Cereal 1 has more, which is good.
Protein, grams	12	9.8	
Salt, grams	0.3	0.03	Cereal 2 scores well. (But this isn't an issue for calorie balance.)

Of course, when choosing which breakfast cereal you will have, taste also comes into it, but I would suggest that you can immediately see quite a saving in energy intake by choosing one over the other. The greater fibre content in cereal 1 is also potentially helpful, as we saw in Chapter 11: remember that we are recommended to take 30 grams of fibre every day.

We are recommended to take no more than 6 grams of salt per day to help our blood pressure. But, on average, working-age adults in England consume 8.4 grams each day.[4] Both these cereals are low in salt. Other packaged foods may not be. For example, a bag of crisps (potato chips in the USA) that I have to hand has 3 grams of salt per 100 grams, and although the pack suggests that a typical portion might be 38 grams, containing 1.11 grams of salt, I must say that I might find it difficult to stop there.

Front-of-pack labelling

In the EU and UK, there is also front-of-pack labelling, which is not mandatory, although all leading retailers now include this. This mostly involves a 'traffic light' system where red indicates a food high in a particular component, green low, and amber intermediate. It's easy to see and helpful for a quick glance, but I would suggest that once you get used to reading the back-of-pack labelling, you will get more information that way.

Ingredients list

There is also mandatory listing of ingredients in a specified format. This is useful to the consumer with an interest in what they are eating (other than taste and cost). When looking at ultra-processed foods in Chapter 11, I noted that these tend to have long lists of ingredients. Sticking with breakfast cereals for continuity, I will just contrast the ingredients list for porridge oats (simply '100% rolled oat flakes') with that for another cereal (cereal 2 in the table above):

Wholegrain oat flakes (56%), golden syrup (*partially inverted sugar syrup*), barley flakes, *vegetable oil* (rapeseed and sunflower in varying proportions), dark chocolate curls (4.5%) (cocoa solids: 70% minimum (cocoa mass, sugar, cocoa butter, emulsifier (soya lecithin), natural flavouring)), freeze dried sliced cherries (3%), macadamia nuts (2.5%), cocoa powder (2%), sunflower seeds.

The porridge oats would count as 'minimally processed', and provide 374 kcal per 100 grams, with 9 grams of fibre, whereas the other cereal is a typical ultra-processed food and provides 441 kcal per 100 grams, with less fibre, as in the table. You can see that this is not the sort of food my grandmother would have made; it looks more like something concocted in a food laboratory. It's clearly been designed to taste good and make you want to eat more.

With regard to calorie balance, I would suggest that the most useful information is the energy content, on the nutrition label, and that the list of ingredients can alert you to added sugars and fats – both increasing the energy density of the food. See the items in italics in the list above.

Acknowledgements

Many people have helped me with this book. My family and friends have been test-readers (and only too ready to point out where my ingrained scientist style made reading difficult): thanks, Theresa, Liz, Nick, Rayya, Alastair (also for information on athletes), Jibreel, Dan, Laith, Susan and Neil. I have talked to many experts while working on the text, who in return have supplied useful information and sent me papers and reports that I should have read, including Barbara Fielding, Jim Hill, Leanne Hodson, Susan Jebb, Fredrik Karpe, Ian Macdonald, Joe Millward, Ann Prentice, Eric Ravussin, Dan Rosoff, Mike Symonds, Sara Stanner and Graham Tobin. Grateful thanks to Sara Stanner and the team at the British Nutrition Foundation who spent time helping me with many aspects of nutrition and labelling, and Sara especially for reading sections and advising on the 'Evidence-based eating' chapter. Ruth Harris and Graham Tobin sent information on obesity physiologist Romaine Hervey. Margaret Ashworth was especially helpful over Elsie Widdowson and Robert McCance, and was the source of the photo of them in the Lake District. Fredrik Karpe, Alan Garrow, Chris Zender, Victor Choules, Michael Goran and Charles Young have kindly given me permission to quote from them or write about them or, in Alan's case, write about his father John. Despite all this help, there will be errors in the text, for which I must take responsibility.

My agent Peter Tallack, in collaboration with Ella Miodownik, was very helpful in sorting out my random thoughts and making them into a well-argued proposal, and Holly Harley at Piatkus was kind enough to take them seriously and offer a contract. Holly has seen through my over-scientific jargon and helped me to write something that I hope will be readable – and interesting. Jan Cutler, who copy-edited the book, and Jillian Stewart, my desk editor at Piatkus, have tidied up my writing and deserve thanks for wading through the whole document in great detail. Thanks also to the wider publishing team in production, marketing and publicity – and to the cover designer.

Finally, thanks most of all to Theresa with whom I have shared most of my adult life, working out together how to keep our lives balanced, as well as our calories.

References

Chapter 1

1. Lustig, R.H., Sugar: The Bitter Truth, University of California, 2009 https://www.youtube.com/watch?v=dBnniua6-oM&t=151s

2. University of Cambridge, 'Slim people have a genetic advantage when it comes to maintaining their weight', 2019 https://www.cam.ac.uk/research/news/slim-people-have-a-genetic-advantage-when-it-comes-to-maintaining-their-weight

3. Harvard Medical School, 'Is a sluggish metabolism to blame for your weight gain?', 2021 https://www.health.harvard.edu/staying-healthy/the-truth-about-metabolism

4. McKie, D., *Antoine Lavoisier: Scientist, Economist, Social Reformer*, New York: Da Capo Press, 1990

5. Blaxter, K.L., 'Adair Crawford and calorimetry', *Proceedings of the Nutrition Society* 1978;37:1–3

6. Buchholz, A.C., Schoeller, D.A., 'Is a calorie a calorie?', *American Journal of Clinical Nutrition* 2004;79:899S–906S

7. The National Weight Control Registry, http://www.nwcr.ws/

8. Hill, J.O., Wyatt, H.R., Peters, J.C., 'Energy balance and obesity', *Circulation* 2012;126:126–32

9. Flatt, J.P., 'Issues and misconceptions about obesity', *Obesity* 2011;19:676–86

10. United States Department of Agriculture, 'What we eat in America', NHANES 2001–2002 https://www.ars.usda.gov/ARSUserFiles/80400530/pdf/0102/Table_1_BIA.pdf

11. United States Department of Agriculture, 'What we eat in America', NHANES 2017–2018 https://www.ars.usda.gov/ARSUserFiles/80400530/pdf/1718/Table_5_EIN_GEN_17.pdf

12. Schiller, J.S., Clarke, T.C., Norris, T., 'Early release of selected estimates based on data from the January–September 2017 National Health Interview Survey', 2018 https://www.cdc.gov/nchs/data/nhis/earlyrelease/earlyrelease201803.pdf

13. Centers for Disease Control and Prevention, 'Adult Obesity Facts', 2022 https://www.cdc.gov/obesity/php/data-research/adult-obesity-facts.html?CDC_AAref_Val=https://www.cdc.gov/obesity/data/adult.html

14. Public Health England, 'NDNS: Results from years 9 to 11 (2016 to 2017 and 2018 to 2019)', 2020 https://www.gov.uk/government/statistics/ndns-results-from-years-9-to-11-2016-to-2017-and-2018-to-2019

15. Sport England, 'Active Lives Adult Survey', November 2020–21 Report, 2022 https://sportengland-production-files.s3.eu-west-2.amazonaws.com/s3fs-public/2022-04/Active%20Lives%20Adult%20Survey%20November%2020-21%20Report.pdf?VersionId=nPU_v3jFjwG8o_xnv62FcKOdEiVmRWCb

16. Moody, A., for NHS Digital, 'Health Survey for England 2019: Overweight and obesity in adults and children', 2020 https://files.digital.nhs.uk/9D/4195D5/HSE19-Overweight-obesity-rep.pdf

17. NCD Risk Factor Collaboration, 'Worldwide trends in underweight and obesity from 1990 to 2022: A pooled analysis of 3663 population representative studies with 222 million children, adolescents, and adults', *Lancet* 2024; http://dx.doi.org/10.1016/S0140-6736(23)02750-2

18. Ludwig, D.S., Aronne, L.J., Astrup, A., et al., 'The carbohydrate-insulin model: A physiological perspective on the obesity pandemic', *American Journal of Clinical Nutrition* 2021;114:1873–85

19. Taubes, G., 'The science of obesity: What do we really know about what makes us fat?', *British Medical Journal* 2013;346:f1050

20. Lustig, R.H., Collier, D., Kassotis, C., et al., 'Obesity I: Overview and molecular and biochemical mechanisms', *Biochemical Pharmacology* 2022;199:115012

21. Atkinson, R.L., 'Could viruses contribute to the worldwide epidemic of obesity?', *International Journal of Pediatric Obesity* 2008;3 Suppl 1:37–43

22. Clay, R.A., 'More than one way to measure', American

Psychological Association, 2010 https://www.apa.org/monitor/2010/09/trials

23. Cena, H., Calder, P.C., 'Defining a healthy diet: Evidence for the role of contemporary dietary patterns in health and disease', *Nutrients* 2020;12 334; doi:10.3390/nu12020334

24. Gao, M., Jebb, S.A., Aveyard, P., et al., 'Associations between dietary patterns and the incidence of total and fatal cardiovascular disease and all-cause mortality in 116,806 individuals from the UK Biobank: A prospective cohort study', *BMC Medicine* 2021;19:83

25. British Nutrition Foundation, 'A healthy, balanced diet', 2023 https://www.nutrition.org.uk/healthy-sustainable-diets/healthy-and-sustainable-diets/a-healthy-balanced-diet/

Chapter 2

1. Kaiyala, K.J., Ramsay, D.S., 'Direct animal calorimetry: The underused gold standard for quantifying the fire of life', *Comparative Biochemistry and Physiology Part A: Molecular & Integrative Physiology* 2011;158:252–64

2. Schoeller, D.A., van Santen, E., 'Measurement of energy expenditure in humans by doubly labeled water method', *Journal of Applied Physiology: Respiratory, Environmental and Exercise Physiology* 1982;53:955–9

3. Frayn, K.N., *Understanding Human Metabolism*, Cambridge: CUP, 2022

4. Heymsfield, S.B., Bourgeois, B., Thomas, D.M., 'Assessment of human energy exchange: Historical overview', *European Journal of Clinical Nutrition* 2017;71:294–300

5. Wilder, R.M., 'Calorimetry: The basis of the science of nutrition', *Archives of Internal Medicine* 1959;103:146–54; Durnin, J.V.G.A., Passmore, R., *Energy, Work and Leisure*, London: Heinemann Educational Books, 1967

6. Trout, D.L., 'Max Josef von Pettenkofer (1818–1901): A biographical sketch', *Journal of Nutrition* 1977;107:1567–74

7. Heymsfield, S.B., Bourgeois, B., Thomas, D.M., 'Assessment of human energy exchange: Historical overview', *European Journal of Clinical Nutrition* 2017;71:294–300; Chambers, W.H., 'Max Rubner: June 2, 1854–April 27, 1932', *Journal of Nutrition* 1952;48:3–12

8. Chambers, W.H., 'Max Rubner: June 2, 1854–April 27, 1932', *Journal of Nutrition* 1952;48:3–12

9. Carpenter, K.J., 'The 1993 W.O. Atwater Centennial Memorial Lecture: The life and times of W.O. Atwater (1844–1907)', *Journal of Nutrition* 1994;124:1707S–14S

10. Atwater, W.O., Rosa, E.B., 'A new respiration calorimeter and experiments on the conservation of energy in the human body, 1', *The Physical Review* 1899;IX:129–66

11. Atwater, W.O., Benedict', F.G., 'The respiration calorimeter', *Yearbook of the Department of Agriculture* 1904:205–20

12. Atwater, W.O., Rosa, E.B., 'A new respiration calorimeter and experiments on the conservation of energy in the human body, 1', *The Physical Review* 1899;IX:129–66

13. Frayn, K.N., *Understanding Human Metabolism*, Cambridge: CUP, 2022; Benedict, F.G., *A Study of Prolonged Fasting*, Washington DC: Carnegie Institute of Washington, 1915

14. Atwater, W.O., Benedict, F.G., 'Experiments on the metabolism of matter and energy in the human body 1900–1902', Washington DC: United States Department of Agriculture, 1903

15. Merrill, A.L., Watt, B.K., 'Energy value of foods: Basis and derivation', Washington, DC: Agricultural Research Service, US Department of Agriculture, 1973

16. Atwater, W.O., Rosa, E.B., 'A new respiration calorimeter and experiments on the conservation of energy in the human body, 1', *The Physical Review* 1899;IX:129–66

17. Atwater, W.O., Benedict F.G., 'The respiration calorimeter', *Yearbook of the Department of Agriculture* 1904:205–20

18. Atwater, W.O., Benedict, F.G., 'Experiments on the metabolism of matter and energy in the human body 1900–1902', Washington DC: United States Department of Agriculture, 1903, see Table 107

19. Atwater, W.O., Benedict, F.G., 'A respiration calorimeter with appliances for the direct determination of oxygen', Washington DC: 1905, see Table 14

20. Atwater, W.O., Benedict, F.G., 'A respiration calorimeter with appliances for the direct determination of oxygen', Washington DC: 1905, see Table 15

21. Atwater, W.O., 'Principles of nutrition and nutritive value of food', Washington DC: US Department of Agriculture, 1902, see Table II

22. Widdowson, E.M., 'Assessment of the energy value of human foods', *Proceedings of the Nutrition Society* 1955;14:142–54

23. Atwater, W.O., 'The chemical composition of American food materials', Washington DC: US Department of Agriculture, 1906

24. Widdowson, E.M., 'Assessment of the energy value of human foods', *Proceedings of the Nutrition Society* 1955;14:142–54

25. Hervey, G.R., 'Control of appetite: Personal and departmental recollections', *Appetite* 2013;61:100–110; Widdowson, E.M., 'R.A. McCance (9 December 1898–5 March 1993)', *Proceedings of the Nutrition Society* 1993;52:383–6

26. Public Health England, 'McCance and Widdowson's "composition of foods integrated dataset" on the nutrient content of the UK food supply', 2021 https://www.gov.uk/government/publications/composition-of-foods-integrated-dataset-cofid

27. Ashwell, M., 'Elsie Widdowson (1906–2000)', *Nature* 2000;406:844

28. Keys, A., Brozek, J., Henschel, A., Mickelsen, O., Taylor, H.L., *The Biology of Human Starvation* (2 vols), Minneapolis: University of Minnesota Press, 1950

29. Ashwell, M., 'Elsie Widdowson (1906–2000)', *Nature* 2000;406:844; Ashwell, M., ed., *McCance & Widdowson: A Scientific Partnership of 60 Years*, London: British Nutrition Foundation, 1993

30. Ashwell, M., ed., *McCance & Widdowson: A Scientific Partnership of 60 Years*, London: British Nutrition Foundation, 1993

31. W.S., and A.R.M., 'Reginald Passmore (Obituary)', *Proceedings of the Royal College of Physicians of Edinburgh* 1999;29:358–62

32. Passmore, R., Thomson, J.G., Warnock, G.M., et al., 'A balance sheet of the estimation of energy intake and energy expenditure as measured by indirect calorimetry, using the Kofranyi-Michaelis calorimeter', *British Journal of Nutrition* 1952;6:253–64

33. Taggart, N., 'Diet, activity and body-weight: A study of variations in a woman', *British Journal of Nutrition* 1962;16:223–35

34. Frayn, K.N., *Understanding Human Metabolism*, Cambridge: CUP, 2022

35. Oxford BioBank, https://www.oxfordbiobank.org.uk/

36. Garrow, J.S., *Energy Balance and Obesity in Man*,

Amsterdam, London: North-Holland Publishing Co., 1974, see p. 43, Fig. 2.2

37. Passmore, R., 'Energy balances in man', *Proceedings of the Nutrition Society* 1967;26:97–101

Chapter 3

1. Ashwell, M., ed., *McCance & Widdowson: A Scientific Partnership of 60 Years*, London: British Nutrition Foundation, 1993

2. Royal College of Physicians, Otto Gustaf Edholm, https://history.rcplondon.ac.uk/inspiring-physicians/otto-gustaf-edholm; K.J.C., 'Obituary: Otto Gustav Edholm', *Annals of Human Biology* 1985;12:383–4

3. Widdowson, E.M., Edholm, O.G., McCance, R.A., 'The food intake and energy expenditure of cadets in training', *British Journal of Nutrition* 1954;8:147–55

4. Ashwell, M., ed., *McCance & Widdowson: A Scientific Partnership of 60 Years*, London: British Nutrition Foundation, 1993

5. Edholm, O.G., Fletcher, J.G., Widdowson, E.M., McCance, R.A., 'The energy expenditure and food intake of individual men', *British Journal of Nutrition* 1955;9:286–300

6. Durnin, J.V., '"Appetite" and the relationships between expenditure and intake of calories in man', *The Journal of Physiology* 1961;156:294–306

7. Edholm, O.G., Adam, J.M., Healy, M.J., Wolff, H.S., Goldsmith, R., Best, T.W., 'Food intake and energy expenditure of army recruits', *British Journal of Nutrition* 1970;24:1091–107

8. Durnin, J.V., Edholm, O.G., Miller, D.S., Waterlow, J.C., 'How much food does man require?', *Nature* 1973;242:418

9. Centers for Disease Control and Prevention, 'About the National Health and Nutrition Examination Survey', https://www.cdc.gov/nchs/nhanes/about_nhanes.htm

10. Centers for Disease Control and Prevention, 'Measuring Guides for the Dietary Recall Interview', https://www.cdc.gov/nchs/nhanes/measuring_guides_dri/measuringguides.htm

11. Public Health England, 'Evaluation of changes in the dietary methodology in the National Diet and Nutrition Survey Rolling Programme from Year 12 (2019 to 2020) Stage 1', London: Public Health England, 2021

12. Black, A.E., Goldberg, G.R., Jebb, S.A., Livingstone, M.B., Cole, T.J., Prentice, A.M., 'Critical evaluation of energy intake data using fundamental principles of energy physiology: 2. Evaluating the results of published surveys', *European Journal of Clinical Nutrition* 1991;45:583–99

13. Ibid.

14. Hallfrisch, J., Steele, P., Cohen, L., 'Comparison of seven-day diet record with measured food intake of twenty-four subjects', *Nutrition Research* 1982;2:263–73; Mertz, W., Tsui, J.C., Judd, J.T., et al., 'What are people really eating? The relation between energy intake derived from estimated diet records and intake determined to maintain body weight', *American Journal of Clinical Nutrition* 1991;54:291–5

15. Livingstone, M.B., Black, A.E., 'Markers of the validity of reported energy intake', *Journal of Nutrition* 2003;133 Suppl 3:895S–920S

16. Murakami, K., Livingstone, M.B., 'Prevalence and characteristics of misreporting of energy intake in US children and adolescents: National Health and Nutrition Examination Survey (NHANES) 2003–2012', *British Journal of Nutrition* 2016;115:294–304

17. Ho, D.K.N., Tseng, S.H., Wu, M.C., et al., 'Validity of image-based dietary assessment methods: A systematic review and meta-analysis', *Clinical Nutrition* 2020;39:2945–59

18. Burrows, T.L., Ho, Y.Y., Rollo, M.E., Collins, C.E., 'Validity of dietary assessment methods when compared to the method of doubly labelled water: A systematic review in adults', *Frontiers in Endocrinology* 2019;10:850

Chapter 4

1. Frayn, K.N., Evans, R.D., *Human Metabolism: a Regulatory Perspective*, 4th edn, Hoboken, NJ: Wiley-Blackwell, 2019

2. Ibid.

3. Wakil, S.J., Pugh, E.L., Sauer, F., 'The mechanism of fatty acid synthesis', *Proceedings of the National Academy of Sciences USA* 1964;52:106–14

4. Frayn, K.N., 'The glucose-fatty acid cycle: A physiological perspective', *Biochemical Society Transactions* 2003;31:1115–19

Chapter 5

1. Garrow, J.S., *Energy Balance and Obesity in Man*, 2nd edn, Amsterdam, New York, Oxford: Elsevier/North Holland Biomedical Press, 1978; Garrow, J.S., Stalley, S., 'Is there a "set point" for human body weight?', *Proceedings of the Nutrition Society* 1975;34:84A–5A; Garrow, J.S., Stalley, S., 'Cognitive thresholds and human body weight', *Proceedings of the Nutrition Society* 1977;36:18A

2. Garrow, J.S., personal communication, 2004

3. Garrow, J.S., Stalley, S., 'Cognitive thresholds and human body weight', *Proceedings of the Nutrition Society* 1977;36:18A

4. Ibid.

5. King, B.M., 'The rise, fall, and resurrection of the ventromedial hypothalamus in the regulation of feeding behavior and body weight', *Physiology & Behavior* 2006;87:221–44

6. Sills, E.S., Vrbikova, J., Kastratovic-Kotlica, B., 'Conjoined twins, conception, pregnancy, and delivery: A reproductive history of the pygopagus Blazek sisters (1878–1922)', *American Journal of Obstetrics and Gynecology* 2001;185:1396–402

7. Hervey, G.R., 'Conjoined twins', *Journal of the Royal Society of Medicine* 2005;98:295–6

8. Hervey, G.R., 'Control of appetite: Personal and departmental recollections', *Appetite* 2013;61:100–110

9. Hervey, G.R., 'The effects of lesions in the hypothalamus in parabiotic rats', *Journal of Physiology* 1959;145:336–52

10. Pool, R., *Fat. Fighting the Obesity Epidemic*, New York: Oxford University Press Inc., 2001

11. Coleman, D.L., 'Obese and diabetes: Two mutant genes causing diabetes-obesity syndromes in mice', *Diabetologia* 1978;14:141–8

12. Zhang, Y., Proenca, R., Maffei, M., Barone, M., Leopold, L., Friedman, J.M., 'Positional cloning of the mouse *obese* gene and its human homologue', *Nature* 1994;372:425–32

13. Considine, R.V., Sinha, M.K., Heiman, M.L., et al., 'Serum immunoreactive-leptin concentrations in normal-weight and obese humans', *New England Journal of Medicine* 1996;334:292–5

14. Pool, R., *Fat. Fighting the Obesity Epidemic*, New York: Oxford University Press Inc., 2001

15. Gura, T., 'Obesity research: Leptin not impressive in clinical trial', *Science* 1999;286:881–2

16. Izquierdo, A.G., Crujeiras, A.B., Casanueva, F.F., Carreira, M.C., 'Leptin, obesity, and leptin resistance: Where are we 25 years later?', *Nutrients* 2019;11

17. Friedman, J.M., 'Leptin and the endocrine control of energy balance', *Nature Metabolism* 2019;1:754–64

18. Montague, C.T., Farooqi, I.S., Whitehead, J.P., et al., 'Congenital leptin deficiency is associated with severe early-onset obesity in humans', *Nature* 1997;387:903–8

19. Farooqi, I.S., Matarese, G., Lord, G.M., et al., 'Beneficial effects of leptin on obesity, T cell hyporesponsiveness, and neuroendocrine/metabolic dysfunction of human congenital leptin deficiency', *Journal of Clinical Investigation* 2002;110:1093–103

20. Licinio, J., Caglayan, S., Ozata, M., et al., 'Phenotypic effects of leptin replacement on morbid obesity, diabetes mellitus, hypogonadism, and behavior in leptin-deficient adults', *Proceedings of the National Academy of Sciences USA* 2004;101:4531–6

21. Stunkard, A.J., Harris, J.R., Pedersen, N.L., McClearn, G.E., 'The body-mass index of twins who have been reared apart', *New England Journal of Medicine* 1990;322:1483–7; Stunkard, A.J., Sørensen, T.I.A., Hanis, C., et al., 'An adoption study of human obesity', *New England Journal of Medicine* 1986;314:193–8

22. 'Genetics of Obesity Study', https://www.goos.org.uk/about-us/what-have-we-discovered

23. Goodarzi, M.O., 'Genetics of obesity: What genetic association studies have taught us about the biology of obesity and its complications', *Lancet Diabetes & Endocrinology* 2018;6:223–36

24. Yeo, G.S., 'The role of the FTO (Fat Mass and Obesity Related) locus in regulating body size and composition', *Molecular and Cellular Endocrinology* 2014;397:34–41

25. Laber, S., Forcisi, S., Bentley, L., et al., 'Linking the FTO obesity rs1421085 variant circuitry to cellular, metabolic, and organismal phenotypes in vivo', *Science Advances* 2021;7

26. Drucker, D.J., 'GLP-1 physiology informs the pharmacotherapy of obesity', *Molecular Metabolism* 2022;57:101351

27. Lustig, R.H., Collier, D., Kassotis, C., et al., 'Obesity I:

Overview and molecular and biochemical mechanisms',
Biochemical Pharmacology 2022;199:115012

Chapter 6

1. Frayn, K.N., Little, R.A., Stoner, H.B., 'Metabolic control
   in non-septic patients with musculoskeletal injuries', *Injury*
   1984;16:73–9
2. Cannon, B., Nedergaard, J., 'Brown adipose tissue: Function
   and physiological significance', *Physiological Reviews*
   2004;84:277–359
3. Nedergaard, J., Bengtsson, T., Cannon, B., 'Unexpected
   evidence for active brown adipose tissue in adult humans',
   *American Journal of Physiology: Endocrinology and
   Metabolism* 2007;293:E444–52
4. Virtanen, K.A., Lidell, M.E., Orava, J., et al., 'Functional
   brown adipose tissue in healthy adults', *New England Journal
   of Medicine* 2009;360:1518–25
5. van der Lans, A.A., Hoeks, J., Brans, B., et al., 'Cold
   acclimation recruits human brown fat and increases
   nonshivering thermogenesis', *Journal of Clinical Investigation*
   2013;123:3395–403
6. Warwick, P.M., Busby, R., 'Influence of mild cold on 24 h
   energy expenditure in "normally" clothed adults', *British
   Journal of Nutrition* 1990;63:481–8
7. van Marken Lichtenbelt, W.D., Vanhommerig, J.W.,
   Smulders, N.M., et al., 'Cold-activated brown adipose
   tissue in healthy men', *New England Journal of Medicine*
   2009;360:1500–508
8. Marlatt, K.L., Ravussin, E., 'Brown adipose tissue: An update
   on recent findings', *Current Obesity Reports* 2017;6:389–96
9. Cypess, A.M., 'Reassessing human adipose tissue', *New
   England Journal of Medicine* 2022;386:768–79
10. Kowaltowski, A.J., 'Cold exposure and the metabolism
    of mice, men, and other wonderful creatures', *Physiology*
    2022;37:253–9
11. Marlatt, K.L., Ravussin, E., 'Brown adipose tissue: An update
    on recent findings', *Current Obesity Reports* 2017;6:389–96
12. Kowaltowski, A.J., 'Cold exposure and the metabolism
    of mice, men, and other wonderful creatures', *Physiology*
    2022;37:253–9
13. Cypess, A.M., Weiner, L.S., Roberts-Toler, C., et al.,

'Activation of human brown adipose tissue by a β3-adrenergic receptor agonist', *Cell Metabolism* 2015;21:33–8

14. Rothwell, N.J., Stock, M.J., 'A role for brown adipose tissue in diet-induced thermogenesis', *Nature* 1979;281:31–5

15. Sims, E.A., 'Experimental obesity, dietary-induced thermogenesis, and their clinical implications', *Clinical Endocrinology and Metabolism* 1976;5:377–95

16. Pasquet, P., Brigant, L., Froment, A., et al., 'Massive overfeeding and energy balance in men: The *Guru Walla* model', *American Journal of Clinical Nutrition* 1992;56:483–90

17. A couple of years before this, Mike had agreed to be the PhD examiner for a young surgeon, Jas Samra, studying fat metabolism in my laboratory. Shortly before the oral examination, which would by convention be held in Oxford, Mike contacted me to say that there was a small problem: he was going into hospital to have a lung removed. 'But if you can arrange for the examination to be held at my bedside [in London], we can still go ahead,' he said. And so it was, and as usual Mike was a thorough but kind examiner – and Jas is now a senior surgeon in Australia.

18. Stock, M.J., 'Gluttony and thermogenesis revisited', *International Journal of Obesity* 1999;23:1105–17

19. Bray, G.A., 'In the footsteps of Wilbur Olin Atwater: The Atwater Lecture for 2019', *Advances in Nutrition* 2020;11:743–50

20. Johannsen, D.L., Marlatt, K.L., Conley, K.E., Smith, S.R., Ravussin, E., 'Metabolic adaptation is not observed after 8 weeks of overfeeding but energy expenditure variability is associated with weight recovery', *American Journal of Clinical Nutrition* 2019;110:805–13

21. Levine, J.A., 'Transform 2010', https://www.youtube.com/watch?v=S6eIvxqaezE

22. Levine, J.A., Eberhardt, N.L., Jensen, M.D., 'Role of nonexercise activity thermogenesis in resistance to fat gain in humans', *Science* 1999;283:212–14

23. When I met Levine on a visit to the Mayo Clinic, he was standing at his specially built desk, working at his computer. I had been invited to the Mayo Clinic by the physician-scientist Mike Jensen, a co-author with Levine on the overfeeding study.

24. Rose, G.A., Williams, R.T., 'Metabolic studies on large and small eaters', *British Journal of Nutrition* 1961;15:1–9

25. McNeill, G., McBride, A., Smith, J.S., James, W.P.T., 'Energy expenditure in large and small eaters', *Nutrition Research* 1989;9:363–72

26. George, V., Tremblay, A., Després, J.-P., et al., 'Further evidence for the presence of "small eaters" and "large eaters" among women', *American Journal of Clinical Nutrition* 1991;53:425–9

27. Clark, D., Tomas, F., Withers, R.T., et al., 'Differences in energy metabolism between normal weight "large-eating" and "small-eating" women', *British Journal of Nutrition* 1992;68:31–44

28. Clark, D., Tomas, F., Withers, R.T., et al., 'No major differences in energy metabolism between matched and unmatched groups of "large-eating" and "small-eating" men', *British Journal of Nutrition* 1993;70:393–406

29. Clark, D., Tomas, F., Withers, R.T., et al., 'Energy metabolism in free-living, "large-eating" and "small-eating" women: Studies using $^2H_2^{18}O$', *British Journal of Nutrition* 1994;72:21–31

30. Bathalon, G.P., Hays, N.P., McCrory, M.A., et al., 'The energy expenditure of postmenopausal women classified as restrained or unrestrained eaters', *European Journal of Clinical Nutrition* 2001;55:1059–67

31. Verboeket-van de Venne, W.P., Westerterp, K.R., ten Hoor, F., 'Substrate utilization in man: Effects of dietary fat and carbohydrate', *Metabolism* 1994;43:152–6; Lawson, O.J., Williamson, D.A., Champagne, C.M., et al., 'The association of body weight, dietary intake, and energy expenditure with dietary restraint and disinhibition', *Obesity Research* 1995;3:153–61

32. Tuschl, R.J., Platte, P., Laessle, R.G., Stichler, W., Pirke, K.M., 'Energy expenditure and everyday eating behavior in healthy young women', *American Journal of Clinical Nutrition* 1990;52:81–6

33. Diaz, E., Vasquez-Velasquez, L., 'Energy expenditure and everyday eating behavior in healthy young women (Response to Tuschl *et al.*)', *American Journal of Clinical Nutrition* 1991;53:800–801

34. Platte, P., Wurmser, H., Wade, S.E., Mercheril, A., Pirke, K.M., 'Resting metabolic rate and diet-induced thermogenesis

in restrained and unrestrained eaters', *International Journal of Eating Disorders* 1996;20:33–41

Chapter 7

1. Conard, N.J., 'A female figurine from the basal Aurignacian of Hohle Fels Cave in southwestern Germany', *Nature* 2009;459:248–52
2. Haslam, D., Rigby, N., 'A long look at obesity', *Lancet* 2010;376:85–6
3. Short, T., *A Discourse Concerning the Causes and Effects of Corpulency: Together with the Method for its Prevention and Cure*, 2nd edn, London: J. Roberts, 1728
4. World Health Organization, https://www.who.int/news-room/fact-sheets/detail/obesity-and-overweight
5. Durnin, J.V.G.A., Womersley, J., 'Body fat assessed from total body density and its estimation from skinfold thickness: Measurements on 481 men and women aged from 16 to 72 years', *British Journal of Nutrition* 1974;32:77–97
6. Manolopoulos, K.N., Karpe, F., Frayn, K.N., 'Gluteofemoral body fat as a determinant of metabolic health', *International Journal of Obesity* 2010;34:949–59
7. Haslam, D., Rigby, N., 'A long look at obesity', *Lancet* 2010;376:85–6
8. Papavramidou, N., Christopoulou-Aletra, H., 'Greco-Roman and Byzantine views on obesity', *Obesity Surgery* 2007;17:112–16
9. Abdel-Halim, R.E., 'Obesity: 1000 years ago', *Lancet* 2005;366:204
10. Pepys, S., *The Diary of Samuel Pepys*, 1660, https://www.pepysdiary.com/diary/1660/11/01/
11. Lincoln, J.E., 'Calorie intake, obesity, and physical activity', *American Journal of Clinical Nutrition* 1972;25:390–94
12. Himms-Hagen, J., 'Obesity may be due to a malfunctioning of brown fat', *Canadian Medical Association Journal* 1979;121:1361–4
13. De Luise, M., Blackburn, G.L., Flier, J.S., 'Reduced activity of the red-cell sodium-potassium pump in human obesity', *New England Journal of Medicine* 1980;303:1017–22
14. Keen, H, Thomas, B.J., Jarrett, R.J., Fuller, J.H., 'Nutrient intake, adiposity, and diabetes', *British Medical Journal* 1979;1:655–8

15. Kromhout, D., 'Energy and macronutrient intake in lean and obese middle-aged men (the Zutphen study)', *American Journal of Clinical Nutrition* 1983;37:295–9

16. Pérusse, L., Bouchard, C., Leblanc, C., Tremblay, A., 'Energy intake and physical fitness in children and adults of both sexes', *Nutrition Research* 1984;4:363–70

17. James, W.P., Trayhurn, P., 'An integrated view of the metabolic and genetic basis for obesity', *Lancet* 1976;2:770–73

18. Prentice, A.M., Black, A.E., Coward, W.A., et al., 'High levels of energy expenditure in obese women', *British Medical Journal* 1986;292:983–7

19. Ravussin, E., Burnand, B., Schutz, Y., Jéquier, E., 'Twenty-four-hour energy expenditure and resting metabolic rate in obese, moderately obese, and control subjects', *American Journal of Clinical Nutrition* 1982;35:566–73

20. Garrow, J.S., Webster, J., 'Are pre-obese people energy thrifty?' *Lancet* 1985;1:670–71

21. Seidell, J.C., Muller, D.C., Sorkin, J.D., Andres, R., 'Fasting respiratory exchange ratio and resting metabolic rate as predictors of weight gain: The Baltimore Longitudinal Study on Aging', *International Journal of Obesity* 1992;16:667–74

22. Katzmarzyk, P.T., Pérusse, L., Tremblay, A., Bouchard, C., 'No association between resting metabolic rate or respiratory exchange ratio and subsequent changes in body mass and fatness: 5½ year follow-up of the Québec family study', *European Journal of Clinical Nutrition* 2000;54:610–14

23. Passmore, R., 'The regulation of body-weight in man', *Proceedings of the Nutrition Society* 1971;30:122–7

24. Hall, K.D., Sacks, G., Chandramohan, D., et al., 'Quantification of the effect of energy imbalance on bodyweight', *Lancet* 2011;378:826–37

Chapter 8

1. Stroud, M., *Shadows on the Wasteland*, London: Jonathan Cape, 1993

2. Stroud, M.A., Ritz, P., Coward, W.A., et al., 'Energy expenditure using isotope-labelled water ($^2H_2$$^{18}O$), exercise performance, skeletal muscle enzyme activities and plasma biochemical parameters in humans during 95 days of endurance exercise with inadequate energy intake', *European Journal of Applied Physiology* 1997;76:243–52. Another

interesting scientific aspect of the expedition was that Mike Stroud wanted to measure the rates of turnover of proteins in the body under these extreme conditions. At intervals, each of the two men drank a solution of the amino acid glycine, labelled with a heavy isotope of nitrogen so it could be measured in the laboratory. He collected and stored urine to measure the turnover of proteins. The results showed that rates of synthesis of new proteins were maintained. Mike wrote these results up as a scientific paper and submitted it for publication to the *British Journal of Nutrition*. Since I was then the editor, it landed on my desk. This presented an interesting problem. The journal prided itself upon high standards of statistical analysis, and indeed we had a number of statistical editors to scrutinise newly submitted papers. One thing that the statistical editors regularly picked up was that often studies were based on too few subjects to give generalisable results. In this case, I had to overrule the call for the authors to repeat the experiment on larger numbers of volunteers. Indeed, I looked into this, and discovered that many nutritionists had pioneered experimental work on themselves, a topic I summarised in an editorial (Frayn, K.N., 'Nutritionists as guinea-pigs', *British Journal of Nutrition* 1996;76:157–9) to accompany Mike Stroud's paper in 1996. (This editorial is freely available via Cambridge University Press/*British Journal of Nutrition* should you be interested.)

3. Westerterp, K.R., Kayser, B., Brouns, F., Herry, J.P., Saris, W.H., 'Energy expenditure climbing Mt. Everest', *Journal of Applied Physiology* 1992;73:1815–19

4. Enqvist, J.K., Mattsson, C.M., Johansson, P.H., Brink-Elfegoun, T., Bakkman, L., Ekblom, B.T., 'Energy turnover during 24 hours and 6 days of adventure racing', *Journal of Sports Science* 2010;28:947–55

5. Ainslie, P.N., Campbell, I.T., Frayn, K.N., Humphreys, S.M., Maclaren, D.P.M., Reilly, T., 'Physiological and metabolic responses to a hill walk', *Journal of Applied Physiology* 2002;92:179–87

6. Ainslie, P.N., Campbell, I.T., Frayn, K.N., et al., 'Energy balance, metabolism, hydration, and performance during strenuous hill walking: The effect of age', *Journal of Applied Physiology* 2002;93:714–23

7. Saris, W.H., van Erp-Baart, M.A., Brouns, F., Westerterp,

K.R., ten Hoor, F., 'Study on food intake and energy expenditure during extreme sustained exercise: The Tour de France', *International Journal of Sports Medicine* 1989;10 Suppl 1:S26–31

8. Ibid.
9. Lustig, R.H., 'Sugar: The Bitter Truth', University of California, 2009 https://www.youtube.com/watch?v=dBnniua6-oM&t=151s
10. Siebers, M., Biedermann, S.V., Fuss, J., 'Do endocannabinoids cause the Runner's High? Evidence and open questions', *Neuroscientist* 2023;29:352–69
11. Ainsworth, B.E., 'Compendium of Physical Activities', 2011 https://pacompendium.com/
12. Besson, H., Ekelund, U., Luan, J., et al., 'A cross-sectional analysis of physical activity and obesity indicators in European participants of the EPIC-PANACEA study', *International Journal of Obesity* 2009;33:497–506
13. Bradbury, K.E., Guo, W., Cairns, B.J., Armstrong, M.E., Key, T.J., 'Association between physical activity and body fat percentage, with adjustment for BMI: A large cross-sectional analysis of UK Biobank', *BMJ Open* 2017;7:e011843
14. DiPietro, L., Williamson, D.F., Caspersen, C.J., Eaker, E., 'The descriptive epidemiology of selected physical activities and body weight among adults trying to lose weight: The Behavioral Risk Factor Surveillance System survey 1989', *International Journal of Obesity* 1993;17:69–76
15. Wyatt, H.R., Peters, J.C., Reed, G.W., Barry, M., Hill, J.O., 'A Colorado statewide survey of walking and its relation to excessive weight', *Medicine &Science in Sports & Exercise* 2005;37:724–30
16. Lee, D.C., Pate, R.R., Lavie, C.J., Sui, X., Church, T.S., Blair, S.N., 'Leisure-time running reduces all-cause and cardiovascular mortality risk', *Journal of the American College of Cardiology* 2014;64:472–81
17. Dons, E., Rojas-Rueda, D., Anaya-Boig, E., et al., 'Transport mode choice and body mass index: Cross-sectional and longitudinal evidence from a European-wide study', *Environment International* 2018;119:109–16
18. Walsh, J., Heazlewood, I.T., Climstein, M., 'Body Mass Index in master athletes: Review of the literature', *Journal of Lifestyle Medicine* 2018;8:79–98

19. Celis-Morales, C.A., Lyall, D.M., Petermann, F., et al., 'Do physical activity, commuting mode, cardiorespiratory fitness and sedentary behaviours modify the genetic predisposition to higher BMI? Findings from a UK Biobank study', *International Journal of Obesity* 2019;43:1526–38

20. Maughan, R.J., 'Nutritional aspects of endurance exercise in humans', *Proceedings of the Nutrition Society* 1994;53:181–8

21. Tremblay, A., Després, J.-P., Leblanc, C., et al., 'Effect of intensity of physical activity on body fatness and fat distribution', *American Journal of Clinical Nutrition* 1990;51:153–7; Imbeault, P., Saint-Pierre, S., Almeras, N., Tremblay, A., 'Acute effects of exercise on energy intake and feeding behaviour', *British Journal of Nutrition* 1997;77:511–21

22. Gilliat-Wimberly, M., Manore, M.M., Woolf, K., Swan, P.D., Carroll, S.S., 'Effects of habitual physical activity on the resting metabolic rates and body compositions of women aged 35 to 50 years', *Journal of the American Dietetic Association* 2001;101:1181–8; Westerterp, K.R., Meijer, G.A., Kester, A.D., Wouters, L., ten Hoor, F., 'Fat-free mass as a function of fat mass and habitual activity level', *International Journal of Sports Medicine* 1992;13:163–6

23. Prince, S.A., Adamo, K.B., Hamel, M.E., Hardt, J., Connor Gorber, S., Tremblay, M., 'A comparison of direct versus self-report measures for assessing physical activity in adults: A systematic review', *International Journal of Behavioral Nutrition and Physical Activity* 2008;5:56

24. Westerterp, K.R., 'Exercise, energy expenditure and energy balance, as measured with doubly labelled water', *Proceedings of the Nutrition Society* 2018;77:4–10

25. Saris, W.H., Blair, S.N., van Baak, M.A., et al., 'How much physical activity is enough to prevent unhealthy weight gain? Outcome of the IASO 1st Stock Conference and consensus statement', *Obesity Reviews* 2003;4:101–14

26. Westerterp, K.R., 'Exercise, energy expenditure and energy balance, as measured with doubly labelled water', *Proceedings of the Nutrition Society* 2018;77:4–10

27. Prentice, A.M., Jebb, S.A., 'Obesity in Britain: Gluttony or sloth?' *British Medical Journal* 1995;311:437–9

28. Shaw, K., Gennat, H., O'Rourke, P., Del Mar, C., 'Exercise for overweight or obesity', *Cochrane Database of Systematic Reviews* 2006;2006:CD003817

29. Westerterp, K.R., 'Exercise, energy expenditure and energy balance, as measured with doubly labelled water', *Proceedings of the Nutrition Society* 2018;77:4–10

30. Pontzer, H., Raichlen, D.A., Wood, B.M., Mabulla, A.Z., Racette, S.B., Marlowe, F.W., 'Hunter-gatherer energetics and human obesity', *PLoS One* 2012;7:e40503

31. Pontzer, H., 'Debunking the hunter-gatherer workout', *New York Times*, 2012

32. Turner, J.E., Markovitch, D., Betts, J.A., Thompson, D., 'Nonprescribed physical activity energy expenditure is maintained with structured exercise and implicates a compensatory increase in energy intake', *American Journal of Clinical Nutrition* 2010;92:1009–16

33. Flack, K.D., Ufholz, K., Johnson, L., Fitzgerald, J.S., Roemmich, J.N., 'Energy compensation in response to aerobic exercise training in overweight adults', *American Journal of Physiology: Regulatory, Integrative and Comparative Physiology* 2018;315:R619–R626

34. Stanner, S., Coe, S., eds, *Cardiovascular Disease. Diet, Nutrition and Emerging Risk Factors*, Hoboken, NJ and Chichester: Wiley-Blackwell, 2019

35. Bull, F.C., Al-Ansari, S.S., Biddle, S., et al., 'World Health Organization 2020 guidelines on physical activity and sedentary behaviour', *British Journal of Sports Medicine* 2020;54:1451–62

36. Iso-Markku, P., Kujala, U.M., Knittle, K., Polet, J., Vuoksimaa, E., Waller, K., 'Physical activity as a protective factor for dementia and Alzheimer's disease: Systematic review, meta-analysis and quality assessment of cohort and case-control studies', *British Journal of Sports Medicine* 2022;56:701–9

37. Stensel, D.J., Hardman, A.E., Gill, J.M.R., *Physical Activity and Health: The evidence explained*, 3rd edn, London, New York: Routledge, 2022

Chapter 9

1. Taubes, G., 'The science of obesity: What do we really know about what makes us fat?', *British Medical Journal* 2013;346:f1050

2. Taubes, G., *The Case for Keto*, London: Granta Books, 2020, p36 Kindle edition

3. Ludwig, D.S., Aronne, L.J., Astrup, A., et al., 'The

carbohydrate-insulin model: A physiological perspective on the obesity pandemic', *American Journal of Clinical Nutrition* 2021;114:1873–85

4. Ludwig, D.S., Ebbeling, C.B., 'The Carbohydrate-Insulin Model of obesity: Beyond "calories in, calories out"', *JAMA Internal Medicine* 2018;178:1098–103

5. Astley, C.M., Todd, J.N., Salem, R.M., et al., 'Genetic evidence that carbohydrate-stimulated insulin secretion leads to obesity', *Clinical Chemistry* 2018;64:192–200

6. Ludwig, D.S., Aronne, L.J., Astrup, A., et al., 'The carbohydrate-insulin model: A physiological perspective on the obesity pandemic', *American Journal of Clinical Nutrition* 2021;114:1873–85

7. Flier, J.S., 'Moderating "the great debate": The carbohydrate-insulin vs. the energy balance models of obesity', *Cell Metabolism* 2023;35:737–41

8. Taubes, G., 'The science of obesity: What do we really know about what makes us fat?', *British Medical Journal* 2013;346:f1050

9. Locke, A.E., Kahali, B., Berndt, S.I., et al., 'Genetic studies of body mass index yield new insights for obesity biology', *Nature* 2015;518:197–206

10. Astley, C.M., Todd, J.N., Salem, R.M., et al., 'Genetic evidence that carbohydrate-stimulated insulin secretion leads to obesity', *Clinical Chemistry* 2018;64:192–200

11. Nguyen, A., Khafagy, R., Meerasa, A., Roshandel, D., Paterson, A.D., Dash, S., 'Insulin response to oral glucose and cardiometabolic disease: A Mendelian randomization study to assess potential causality', *Diabetes* 2022;71:1880–90

12. Taubes, G., 'The science of obesity: What do we really know about what makes us fat?', *British Medical Journal* 2013;346:f1050

13. Frayn, K.N., Evans, R.D., *Human Metabolism: a Regulatory Perspective*, 4th edn, Hoboken, NJ: Wiley-Blackwell, 2019

14. The DCCT Research Group, 'Weight gain associated with intensive therapy in the diabetes control and complications trial', *Diabetes Care* 1988;11:567–73

15. Carlson, M.G., Campbell, P.J., 'Intensive insulin therapy and weight gain in IDDM', *Diabetes* 1993;42:1700–707

16. Torbay, N., Bracco, E.F., Geliebter, A., Stewart, I.M., Hashim, S.A., 'Insulin increases body fat despite control of food intake

and physical activity', *American Journal of Physiology: Regulatory, Integrative and Comparative Physiology* 1985;248:R120–24

17. Aaronovitch, D., 'It's time for my fat jab', *The Times Magazine*, 4 Mar 2023

18. Prillaman, M., 'Anti-obesity drugs: What researchers want to know', *Nature* 2023;620:28–30; Campbell, J.E., Muller, T.D., Finan, B., DiMarchi, R.D., Tschop, M.H., D'Alessio, D.A., 'GIPR/GLP-1R dual agonist therapies for diabetes and weight loss-chemistry, physiology, and clinical applications', *Cell Metabolism* 2023;35:1519–29

19. Astrup, A., 'The satiating power of protein: A key to obesity prevention?', *American Journal of Clinical Nutrition* 2005;82:1–2

20. 'thefast800. The new 5:2 diet: intermittent fasting', https:// thefast800.com/the-new-52/

21. Passmore, R., Swindells, Y.E., 'Observations on the respiratory quotients and weight gain', *British Journal of Nutrition* 1963;17:331–9

22. National Institute of Diabetes and Digestive and Kidney Diseases, 'Body Weight Planner: Balancing your food and activity', https://www.niddk.nih.gov/bwp

23. Geissler, C.A., Miller, D.S., Shah, M., 'The daily metabolic rate of the post-obese and the lean', *American Journal of Clinical Nutrition* 1987;45:914–20; Shah, M., Miller, D.S., Geissler, C.A., 'Lower metabolic rates of post-obese versus lean women: Thermogenesis, basal metabolic rate and genetics', *European Journal of Clinical Nutrition* 1988;42:741–52

24. Astrup, A., Gotzsche, P.C., van de Werken, K., et al., 'Meta-analysis of resting metabolic rate in formerly obese subjects', *American Journal of Clinical Nutrition* 1999;69:1117–22

25. Weinsier, R.L., Nelson, K.M., Hensrud, D.D., Darnell, B.E., Hunter, G.R., Schutz, Y., 'Metabolic predictors of obesity: Contribution of resting energy expenditure, thermic effect of food, and fuel utilization to four-year weight gain of post-obese and never-obese women', *Journal of Clinical Investigation* 1995;95:980–85

26. Ostendorf, D.M., Melanson, E.L., Caldwell, A.E., et al., 'No consistent evidence of a disproportionately low resting energy expenditure in long-term successful weight-loss maintainers', *American Journal of Clinical Nutrition* 2018;108:658-66;

Wyatt, H.R., Grunwald, G.K., Seagle, H.M., et al., 'Resting energy expenditure in reduced-obese subjects in the National Weight Control Registry', *American Journal of Clinical Nutrition* 1999;69:1189–93

27. Aronne, L.J., Hall, K.D., Jakicic, J.M., et al., 'Describing the weight-reduced state: Physiology, behavior, and interventions', *Obesity* 2021;29 Suppl 1:S9–S24

28. Martins, C., Dutton, G.R., Hunter, G.R., Gower, B.A., 'Revisiting the Compensatory Theory as an explanatory model for relapse in obesity management', *American Journal of Clinical Nutrition* 2020;112:1170–79; Martins, C., Roekenes, J., Salamati, S., Gower, B.A., Hunter, G.R., 'Metabolic adaptation is an illusion, only present when participants are in negative energy balance', *American Journal of Clinical Nutrition* 2020;112:1212–18

29. WeightWatchers, 'Eat fat to lose fat: What is "good" fat, and how can it help you lose body weight?', 2023 https://www.weightwatchers.com/uk/blog/food/eat-fat-lose-fat-what-good-fat-and-how-can-it-help-you-lose-body-weight

30. Bee, P., 'Lose weight and keep it off: The new rules', *The Times: Times 2*, 11 Apr 2023

31. Doucet, E., Alméras, N., White, M.D., Després, J.-P., Bouchard, C., Tremblay, A., 'Dietary fat composition and human adiposity', *European Journal of Clinical Nutrition* 1998;52:2–6

32. Micallef, M., Munro, I., Phang, M., Garg, M., 'Plasma n-3 polyunsaturated fatty acids are negatively associated with obesity', *British Journal of Nutrition* 2009;102:1370–4

33. Parry, S.A., Rosqvist, F., Cornfield, T., Barrett, A., Hodson, L., 'Oxidation of dietary linoleate occurs to a greater extent than dietary palmitate *in vivo* in humans', *Clinical Nutrition* 2021;40:1108–14

34. Doucet, E., Alméras, N., White, M.D., Després, J.-P., Bouchard, C., Tremblay, A., 'Dietary fat composition and human adiposity', *European Journal of Clinical Nutrition* 1998;52:2–6

35. Bee, P., 'Four weeks to blitz your body: Tone up, trim your waist', *The Times: Saturday Review*, 18 Jun 2022

36. Rai, K., 'Britons told to eat breakfast AFTER 11am in bizarre advice to lose weight "Sheds excess"', 2022 https://www.express.co.uk/news/uk/1624634/

britons-told-eat-breakfast-after-11am-by-nutritionist-tim-spector; Gruffyd, M., 'Dieters should eat breakfast at specific time to lose weight – "lose up to 11 pounds"', 2022 https://www.express.co.uk/life-style/diets/1625266/breakfast-specific-time-of-day-weight-loss-healthy-diet-meal-plan-professor-tim-spector

Chapter 10

1. Atkinson, F.S., Hancock, D., Petocz, P., Brand-Miller, J.C., 'The physiologic and phenotypic significance of variation in human amylase gene copy number', *American Journal of Clinical Nutrition* 2018;108:737–48; Inchley, C.E., Larbey, C.D., Shwan, N.A., et al., 'Selective sweep on human amylase genes postdates the split with Neanderthals', *Science Reports* 2016;6:37198

2. Perry, G.H., Dominy, N.J., Claw, K.G., et al., 'Diet and the evolution of human amylase gene copy number variation', *Nature Genetics* 2007;39:1256–60

3. Santos, J.L., Saus, E., Smalley, S.V., et al., 'Copy number polymorphism of the salivary amylase gene: Implications in human nutrition research', *Journal of Nutrigenetics and Nutrigenomics* 2012;5:117–31

4. Krebs, J.R., 'The gourmet ape: Evolution and human food preferences', *American Journal of Clinical Nutrition* 2009;90:707S–711S

5. Prentice, A.M., 'Fires of life: The struggles of an ancient metabolism in a modern world', *Nutrition Bulletin* 2001;26:13–27

6. Neel, J.V., 'Diabetes mellitus: A "thrifty" genotype rendered detrimental by "progress"?', *American Journal of Human Genetics* 1962;14:353–62

7. Garrow, J.S., *Energy Balance and Obesity in Man*, 2nd edn, Amsterdam, New York, Oxford: Elsevier/North Holland Biomedical Press, 1978, see pp71–2

8. YouGov, '52% of the world's adults are trying to lose weight. Who are they?', https://business.yougov.com/content/44057-52-worlds-adults-trying-lose-weight

9. Benedict, F.G., *A Study of Prolonged Fasting*, Washington DC: Carnegie Institute of Washington, 1915

10. Keys, A., Brozek, J., Henschel, A., Mickelsen, O., Taylor, H.L., *The Biology of Human Starvation* (2 vols), Minneapolis: University of Minnesota Press, 1950

11. Leibel, R.L., Rosenbaum, M., Hirsch, J., 'Changes in energy expenditure resulting from altered body weight', *New England Journal of Medicine* 1995;332:621–8

12. Coleman, R.A., Herrmann, T.S., 'Nutritional regulation of leptin in humans', *Diabetologia* 1999;42:639–46

13. Forbes, G.B., 'Weight loss during fasting: Implications for the obese', *American Journal of Clinical Nutrition* 1970;23:1212–19

14. Barnard, D.L., Ford, J., Garnett, E.S., Mardell, R.J., Whyman, A.E., 'Changes in body composition produced by prolonged total starvation and refeeding', *Metabolism* 1969;18:564–9

15. Diabetes UK, 'Weight loss can put type 2 diabetes into remission for at least 5 years, DiRECT study reveals', 2023 https://www.diabetes.org.uk/about_us/news/ weight-loss-can-put-type-2-diabetes-remission-least-five-years-reveal-latest-findings

16. Taylor, R., Al-Mrabeh, A., Sattar, N., 'Understanding the mechanisms of reversal of type 2 diabetes', *Lancet Diabetes & Endocrinology* 2019;7:726–36

17. Bistrian, B.R., 'Clinical use of a protein-sparing modified fast', *JAMA* 1978;240:2299–302

18. Lean, M.E.J., Leslie, W.S., Barnes, A.C., et al., 'Durability of a primary care-led weight-management intervention for remission of type 2 diabetes: 2-year results of the DiRECT open-label, cluster-randomised trial', *Lancet Diabetes & Endocrinology* 2019;7:344–55

19. Bueno, N.B., de Melo, I.S., de Oliveira, S.L., da Rocha Ataide, T., 'Very-low-carbohydrate ketogenic diet v. low-fat diet for long-term weight loss: A meta-analysis of randomised controlled trials', *British Journal of Nutrition* 2013;110:1178–87; Sackner-Bernstein, J., Kanter, D., Kaul, S., 'Dietary intervention for overweight and obese adults: Comparison of low-carbohydrate and low-fat diets. A meta-analysis', *PLoS One* 2015;10:e0139817; Tobias, D.K., Chen, M., Manson, J.E., Ludwig, D.S., Willett, W., Hu, F.B., 'Effect of low-fat diet interventions versus other diet interventions on long-term weight change in adults: A systematic review and meta-analysis', *Lancet Diabetes & Endocrinology* 2015;3:968–79; Silverii, G.A., Cosentino, C., Santagiuliana, F., et al., 'Effectiveness of low-carbohydrate diets for long-term weight loss in obese individuals: A meta-analysis of randomized

controlled trials', *Diabetes, Obesity and Metabolism* 2022;24:1458–68

20. Silverii, G.A., Cosentino, C., Santagiuliana, F., et al., 'Effectiveness of low-carbohydrate diets for long-term weight loss in obese individuals: A meta-analysis of randomized controlled trials', *Diabetes, Obesity and Metabolism* 2022;24:1458–68; Astrup, A., Meinert Larsen, T., Harper, A., 'Atkins and other low-carbohydrate diets: Hoax or an effective tool for weight loss?', *Lancet* 2004;364:897–9

21. Morris, E., Aveyard, P., Dyson, P., et al., 'A food-based, low-energy, low-carbohydrate diet for people with type 2 diabetes in primary care: A randomized controlled feasibility trial', *Diabetes, Obesity and Metabolism* 2020;22:512–20

22. 'Robert Coleman Atkins: Cardiologist and author of the bestselling diet book in history' [Obituary], *British Medical Journal* 2003;326:1090

23. 'Mayo Clinic Staff. Weight-loss basics', https://www.mayoclinic.org/healthy-lifestyle/weight-loss/basics/weightloss-basics/hlv-20049483; Migala, J., '12 Popular low-carb diets, and their pros and cons', 2023 https://www.everydayhealth.com/diet-nutrition/diet/low-carb-diets-keto-low-carb-paleo-atkins-more/

24. Google search, 2023

25. Noto, H., Goto, A., Tsujimoto, T., Noda, M., 'Low-carbohydrate diets and all-cause mortality: A systematic review and meta-analysis of observational studies', *PLoS One* 2013;8:e55030; Mazidi, M., Katsiki, N., Mikhailidis, D.P., Sattar, N., Banach, M., 'Lower carbohydrate diets and all-cause and cause-specific mortality: A population-based cohort study and pooling of prospective studies', *European Heart Journal* 2019;40:2870–79; Qin, P., Suo, X., Chen, S., et al., 'Low-carbohydrate diet and risk of cardiovascular disease, cardiovascular and all-cause mortality: A systematic review and meta-analysis of cohort studies', *Food & Function* 2023;14:8678–91

26. Seidelmann, S.B., Claggett, B., Cheng, S., et al., 'Dietary carbohydrate intake and mortality: A prospective cohort study and meta-analysis', *Lancet Public Health* 2018;3:e419–e428

27. Taubes, G., *The Case for Keto. The Truth about Low-Carb, High-Fat Eating*, New York: Penguin Random House, 2020

28. Public Health England, 'NDNS: results from years 9 to 11

(2016 to 2017 and 2018 to 2019)', 2020 https://www.gov.uk/government/statistics/ndns-results-from-years-9-to-11-2016-to-2017-and-2018-to-2019

29. Astrup, A., Meinert Larsen, T., Harper, A., 'Atkins and other low-carbohydrate diets: Hoax or an effective tool for weight loss?', *Lancet* 2004;364:897–9

30. Gibson, A.A., Seimon, R.V., Lee, C.M., et al., 'Do ketogenic diets really suppress appetite? A systematic review and meta-analysis', *Obesity Reviews* 2015;16:64–76

31. Astrup, A., Meinert Larsen, T., Harper, A., 'Atkins and other low-carbohydrate diets: Hoax or an effective tool for weight loss?', *Lancet* 2004;364:897–9; Astrup, A., 'The satiating power of protein: A key to obesity prevention?', *American Journal of Clinical Nutrition* 2005;82:1–2

32. Calcagno, M., Kahleova, H., Alwarith, J., et al., 'The thermic effect of food: A review', *Journal of the American College of Nutrition* 2019;38:547–51

33. Astrup, A., Meinert Larsen, T., Harper, A., 'Atkins and other low-carbohydrate diets: Hoax or an effective tool for weight loss?', *Lancet* 2004;364:897–9

34. Ludwig, D.S., Dickinson, S.L., Henschel, B., Ebbeling, C.B., Allison, D.B., 'Do lower-carbohydrate diets increase total energy expenditure? An updated and reanalyzed meta-analysis of 29 controlled-feeding studies', *Journal of Nutrition* 2021;151:482–90; Ebbeling, C.B., Swain, J.F., Feldman, H.A., et al., 'Effects of dietary composition on energy expenditure during weight-loss maintenance', *JAMA* 2012;307:2627–34; Hall, K.D., Chen, K.Y., Guo, J., et al., 'Energy expenditure and body composition changes after an isocaloric ketogenic diet in overweight and obese men', *American Journal of Clinical Nutrition* 2016;104:324–33; The studies I cite here use different settings, such as weight maintenance before or after weight loss. They are also complicated because, as in all dietary studies, if you reduce one component (for example, carbohydrate), you must increase another (for example, protein). The meta-analysis from Ludwig and colleagues discusses these different scenarios.

35. Wheless, J.W., 'History of the ketogenic diet', *Epilepsia* 2008;49 Suppl 8:3–5

36. Kraschnewski, J.L., Boan, J., Esposito, J., et al., 'Long-term

weight loss maintenance in the United States', *International Journal of Obesity* 2010;34:1644–54

37. Hartmann-Boyce, J., Aveyard, P., Jebb, S.A., 'Shedding pounds might benefit your heart even if some weight is regained – new study', The Conversation 2023, https://theconversation.com/shedding-pounds-might-benefit-your-heart-even-if-some-weight-is-regained-new-study-202565; Hartmann-Boyce, J., Theodoulou, A., Oke, J.L., et al., 'Association between characteristics of behavioural weight loss programmes and weight change after programme end: Systematic review and meta-analysis', *BMJ* 2021;374:n1840

38. The National Weight Control Registry, http://www.nwcr.ws/

39. Wing, R.R., Hill, J.O., 'Successful weight loss maintenance', *Annual Review of Nutrition* 2001;21:323–41; Wing, R.R., Phelan, S., 'Long-term weight loss maintenance', *American Journal of Clinical Nutrition* 2005;82:222S–5S

40. Klem, M.L., Wing, R.R., McGuire, M.T., Seagle, H.M., Hill, J.O., 'A descriptive study of individuals successful at long-term maintenance of substantial weight loss', *American Journal of Clinical Nutrition* 1997;66:239–46

41. The National Weight Control Registry, http://www.nwcr.ws/

42. Raynor, D.A., Phelan, S., Hill, J.O., Wing, R.R., 'Television viewing and long-term weight maintenance: Results from the National Weight Control Registry', *Obesity* 2006;14:1816–24

43. Butryn, M.L., Phelan, S., Hill, J.O., Wing, R.R., 'Consistent self-monitoring of weight: A key component of successful weight loss maintenance', *Obesity* 2007;15:3091–6

44. Cassidy, S., Trenell, M., Stefanetti, R.J., et al., 'Physical activity, inactivity and sleep during the Diabetes Remission Clinical Trial (DiRECT)', *Diabetic Medicine* 2023;40:e15010

45. Varkevisser, R.D.M., van Stralen, M.M., Kroeze, W., Ket, J.C.F., Steenhuis, I.H.M., 'Determinants of weight loss maintenance: A systematic review', *Obesity Reviews* 2019;20:171–211

46. Melby, C.L., Paris, H.L., Sayer, R.D., Bell, C., Hill, J.O., 'Increasing energy flux to maintain diet-induced weight loss', *Nutrients* 2019;11

47. Ostendorf, D.M., Lyden, K., Pan, Z., et al., 'Objectively measured physical activity and sedentary behavior in successful weight loss maintainers', *Obesity* 2018;26:53–60

48. Ostendorf, D.M., Caldwell, A.E., Creasy, S.A., et al., 'Physical

activity energy expenditure and total daily energy expenditure in successful weight loss maintainers', *Obesity* 2019;27:496–504

Chapter 11

1. Lissner, L., Levitsky, D.A., Strupp, B.J., Kalkwarf, H.J., Roe, D.A., 'Dietary fat and the regulation of energy intake in human subjects', *American Journal of Clinical Nutrition* 1987;46:886–92

2. Stubbs, R.J., Harbron, C.G., Murgatroyd, P.R., Prentice, A.M., 'Covert manipulation of dietary fat and energy density: Effect on substrate flux and food intake in men eating ad libitum', *American Journal of Clinical Nutrition* 1995;62:316–29

3. Bell, E.A., Rolls, B.J., 'Energy density of foods affects energy intake across multiple levels of fat content in lean and obese women', *American Journal of Clinical Nutrition* 2001;73:1010–18

4. Culling, K.S., Neil, H.A., Gilbert, M., Frayn, K.N., 'Effects of short-term low- and high-carbohydrate diets on postprandial metabolism in non-diabetic and diabetic subjects', *Nutrition, Metabolism and Cardiovascular Diseases* 2009;19:345–51

5. Saquib, N., Natarajan, L., Rock, C.L., et al., 'The impact of a long-term reduction in dietary energy density on body weight within a randomized diet trial', *Nutrition and Cancer* 2008;60:31–8

6. Stelmach-Mardas, M., Rodacki, T., Dobrowolska-Iwanek, J., et al., 'Link between food energy density and body weight changes in obese adults', *Nutrients* 2016;8:229; Rouhani, M.H., Haghighatdoost, F., Surkan, P.J., Azadbakht, L., 'Associations between dietary energy density and obesity: A systematic review and meta-analysis of observational studies', *Nutrition* 2016;32:1037–47

7. Stelmach-Mardas, M., Rodacki, T., Dobrowolska-Iwanek, J., et al., 'Link between food energy density and body weight changes in obese adults', *Nutrients* 2016;8:229; Levine, A.S., 'Energy density of foods: Building a case for food intake management, *American Journal of Clinical Nutrition* 2001;73:999–1000

8. Saquib, N., Natarajan, L., Rock, C.L., et al., 'The impact of a long-term reduction in dietary energy density on body weight within a randomized diet trial', *Nutrition and Cancer* 2008;60:31–8

9. Turley, M.L., Skeaff, C.M., Mann, J.I., Cox, B., 'The effect of a low-fat, high-carbohydrate diet on serum high density lipoprotein cholesterol and triglyceride', *European Journal of Clinical Nutrition* 1998;52:728–32; Saris, W.H., Astrup, A., Prentice, A.M., et al., 'Randomized controlled trial of changes in dietary carbohydrate/fat ratio and simple vs complex carbohydrates on body weight and blood lipids: The CARMEN study. The Carbohydrate Ratio Management in European National diets', *International Journal of Obesity* 2000;24:1310–18; Astrup, A., Grunwald, G.K., Melanson, E.L., Saris, W.H., Hill, J.O., 'The role of low-fat diets in body weight control: A meta-analysis of ad libitum dietary intervention studies', *International Journal of Obesity* 2000;24:1545–52; Poppitt, S.D., Keogh, G.F., Prentice, A.M., et al., 'Long-term effects of ad libitum low-fat, high-carbohydrate diets on body weight and serum lipids in overweight subjects with metabolic syndrome', *American Journal of Clinical Nutrition* 2002;75:11–20

10. World Health Organization, 'Sugars intake for adults and children 2015', https://www.who.int/publications/i/item/9789241549028

11. Public Health England have clarified how this term is to be used: Swan, G.E., Powell, N.A., Knowles, B.L., Bush, M.T., Levy, L.B., 'A definition of free sugars for the UK', *Public Health Nutrition* 2018;21:1636–8

12. Scientific Advisory Committee on Nutrition, *Carbohydrates and Health*, London: The Stationery Office, 2015

13. USDA, 'Dietary Guidelines for Americans 2015–2020. Cut Down on Added Sugars', 2015 https://health.gov/sites/default/files/2019-10/DGA_Cut-Down-On-Added-Sugars.pdf

14. World Health Organization, 'Use of Non-Sugar Sweeteners', 2023 https://www.who.int/publications/i/item/9789240073616

15. Bray, G.A., Nielsen, S.J., Popkin, B.M., 'Consumption of high-fructose corn syrup in beverages may play a role in the epidemic of obesity', *American Journal of Clinical Nutrition* 2004;79:537–43

16. Stanner, S.A., Spiro, A., 'Public health rationale for reducing sugar: Strategies and challenges', *Nutrition Bulletin* 2020;45:253–70

17. Lustig, R.H., 'Sugar: The Bitter Truth', University

of California, 2009 https://www.youtube.com/
watch?v=dBnniua6-oM&t=151s

18. Chong, M.F., Fielding, B.A., Frayn, K.N., 'Mechanisms for
the acute effect of fructose on postprandial lipemia', *American
Journal of Clinical Nutrition* 2007;85:1511–20

19. Scientific Advisory Committee on Nutrition, *Carbohydrates
and Health*, London: The Stationery Office, 2015; Livesey,
G., Taylor, R., Livesey, H.F., et al., 'Dietary glycemic index
and load and the risk of Type 2 diabetes: Assessment of causal
relations', *Nutrients* 2019;11

20. Tappy, L., Rosset, R., 'Health outcomes of a high fructose
intake: The importance of physical activity', *Journal of
Physiology* 2019;597:3561–71

21. Burkitt, D.P., 'Non-infective disease of the large bowel', *British
Medical Bulletin* 1984;40:387–9

22. Ma, Y., Hu, M., Zhou, L., et al., 'Dietary fiber intake and
risks of proximal and distal colon cancers: A meta-analysis',
Medicine (Baltimore) 2018;97:e11678

23. Reynolds, A., Mann, J., Cummings, J., Winter, N., Mete, E.,
Te Morenga, L., 'Carbohydrate quality and human health:
A series of systematic reviews and meta-analyses', *Lancet*
2019;393:434–45

24. Reynolds, A., Mann, J., Cummings, J., Winter, N., Mete, E., Te
Morenga, L., 'Carbohydrate quality and human health: A series
of systematic reviews and meta-analyses', *Lancet* 2019;393:434–
45; Slavin, J.L., 'Dietary fiber and body weight', *Nutrition*
2005;21:411–18; Maskarinec, G., Takata, Y., Pagano, I., et al.,
'Trends and dietary determinants of overweight and obesity in a
multiethnic population', *Obesity* 2006;14:717–26

25. Southgate, D.A., Branch, W.J., Hill, M.J., et al., 'Metabolic
responses to dietary supplements of bran', *Metabolism*
1976;25:1129–35; Wisker, E., Maltz, A., Feldheim, W.,
'Metabolizable energy of diets low or high in dietary fiber
from cereals when eaten by humans', *Journal of Nutrition*
1988;118:945–52

26. Southgate, D.A., Branch, W.J., Hill, M.J., et al., 'Metabolic
responses to dietary supplements of bran', *Metabolism*
1976;25:1129–35

27. Carnero, E.A., Bock, C.P., Liu, Y., et al., 'Measurement of
24-h continuous human CH_4 release in a whole room indirect
calorimeter', *Journal of Applied Physiology* 2023;134:766–76

28. Jenkins, D.J., Jenkins, A.L., 'Dietary fiber and the glycemic response', *Proceedings of the Society for Experimental Biology and Medicine* 1985;180:422–31

29. Blundell, J.E., Green, S., Burley, V., 'Carbohydrates and human appetite', *American Journal of Clinical Nutrition* 1994;59:728S–734S

30. Ohkuma, T., Hirakawa, Y., Nakamura, U., Kiyohara, Y., Kitazono, T., Ninomiya, T., 'Association between eating rate and obesity: A systematic review and meta-analysis', *International Journal of Obesity* 2015;39:1589–96

31. Potter, C., Gibson, E.L., Ferrida, D., et al., 'Associations between number of siblings, birth order, eating rate and adiposity in children and adults', *Clinical Obesity* 2021;11:e12438

32. AnimalSmart.org, 'Why are Antibiotics Used in Animal Production?' https://animalsmart.org/feeding-the-world/antibiotic-use-in-animal-production

33. Kelly, D., Kelly, A., O'Dowd, T., Hayes, C.B., 'Antibiotic use in early childhood and risk of obesity: Longitudinal analysis of a national cohort', *World Journal of Pediatrics* 2019;15:390–97

34. Ley, R.E., Turnbaugh, P.J., Klein, S., Gordon, J.I., 'Microbial ecology: Human gut microbes associated with obesity', *Nature* 2006;444:1022–3

35. Krajmalnik-Brown, R., Ilhan, Z.E., Kang, D.W., DiBaise, J.K., 'Effects of gut microbes on nutrient absorption and energy regulation', *Nutrition in Clinical Practice* 2012;27:201–14

36. Bastos, R.M.C., Simplicio-Filho, A., Savio-Silva, C., et al., 'Fecal microbiota transplant in a pre-clinical model of Type 2 diabetes mellitus, obesity and diabetic kidney disease', *International Journal of Molecular Sciences* 2022;23

37. Hall, K.D., Ayuketah, A., Brychta, R., et al., 'Ultra-processed diets cause excess calorie intake and weight gain: An inpatient randomized controlled trial of ad libitum food intake', *Cell Metabolism* 2019;30:67–77 e3

38. Monteiro, C.A., Cannon, G., Moubarac, J.C., Levy, R.B., Louzada, M.L.C., Jaime, P.C., 'The UN Decade of Nutrition, the NOVA food classification and the trouble with ultra-processing', *Public Health Nutrition* 2018;21:5–17

39. Global Panel on Agriculture and Food Systems for Nutrition,

'Food Systems and Diets: Facing the Challenges of the 21st Century', London: 2016

40. Rauber, F., Louzada, M., Martinez Steele, E., et al., 'Ultra-processed foods and excessive free sugar intake in the UK: A nationally representative cross-sectional study', *BMJ Open* 2019;9:e027546

41. Moubarac, J.C., Martins, A.P., Claro, R.M., Levy, R.B., Cannon, G., Monteiro, C.A., 'Consumption of ultra-processed foods and likely impact on human health: Evidence from Canada', *Public Health Nutrition* 2013;16:2240–48

42. Mosley, M., 'Want to shrink your waistline?', *The Times, Times 2*, 5 Feb 2022; van Tulleken, C., *Ultra-Processed People: Why Do We All Eat Stuff That Isn't Food ... and Why Can't We Stop?* London: Cornerstone Press, 2023

43. Hall, K.D., Ayuketah, A., Brychta, R., et al., 'Ultra-processed diets cause excess calorie intake and weight gain: An inpatient randomized controlled trial of ad libitum food intake', *Cell Metabolism* 2019;30:67–77 e3

44. Pereira, M.A., Kartashov, A.I., Ebbeling, C.B., et al., 'Fast-food habits, weight gain, and insulin resistance (the CARDIA study): 15-year prospective analysis', *Lancet* 2005;365:36–42

45. Schnabel, L., Kesse-Guyot, E., Alles, B., et al., 'Association between ultraprocessed food consumption and risk of mortality among middle-aged adults in France', *JAMA Internal Medicine* 2019;179:490–98; Srour, B., Fezeu, L.K., Kesse-Guyot, E., et al., 'Ultraprocessed food consumption and risk of Type 2 diabetes among participants of the NutriNet-Santé prospective cohort', *JAMA Internal Medicine* 2020;180:283–91; Srour, B., Fezeu, L.K., Kesse-Guyot, E., et al., 'Ultra-processed food intake and risk of cardiovascular disease: Prospective cohort study (NutriNet-Santé)', *BMJ* 2019;365:l1451; Rico-Campà, A., Martínez-González, M.A., Alvarez-Alvarez, I., et al., 'Association between consumption of ultra-processed foods and all cause mortality: SUN prospective cohort study', *BMJ* 2019;365:l1949; Hang, D., Wang, L., Fang, Z., et al., 'Ultra-processed food consumption and risk of colorectal cancer precursors: Results from 3 prospective cohorts', *Journal of the National Cancer Institute* 2023;115:155–64; Pagliai, G., Dinu, M., Madarena, M.P., Bonaccio, M., Iacoviello, L., Sofi, F., 'Consumption of ultra-processed foods and

health status: A systematic review and meta-analysis', *British Journal of Nutrition* 2021;125:308–18

46. Adams, J., White, M., 'Characterisation of UK diets according to degree of food processing and associations with socio-demographics and obesity: Cross-sectional analysis of UK National Diet and Nutrition Survey (2008–12)', *International Journal of Behavioral Nutrition and Physical Activity* 2015;12:160

47. Moubarac, J.C., Martins, A.P., Claro, R.M., Levy, R.B., Cannon, G., Monteiro, C.A., 'Consumption of ultra-processed foods and likely impact on human health: Evidence from Canada', *Public Health Nutrition* 2013;16:2240–48

48. dos Santos Simões, B., de Oliveira Cardoso, L., Benseñor, I.J.M., et al., 'Consumption of ultra-processed foods and socioeconomic position: A cross-sectional analysis of the Brazilian Longitudinal Study of Adult Health (ELSA-Brasil)', *Cadernos de Saúde Pública* 2018;34:e00019717

49. Sellem, L., Srour, B., Javaux, G., et al., 'Food additive emulsifiers and risk of cardiovascular disease in the NutriNet-Santé cohort: Prospective cohort study', *BMJ* 2023;382:e076058

50. Stanner, S., 17 Aug 2023, personal communication

51. British Nutrition Foundation, 'BNF survey reveals confusion about ultra-processed foods', 2021 https://www.nutrition.org.uk/news/2021/bnf-survey-reveals-confusion-about-ultra-processed-foods/

52. British Nutrition Foundation, 'FAQs: Processed food', 2021 https://www.nutrition.org.uk/putting-it-into-practice/make-healthier-choices/perspectives-on-processed-foods/faqs-on-processed-foods/

53. Hayward, E., 'Half-baked idea that beans on toast is unhealthy', *The Times*, 27 Apr 2023

54. Stanner, S., 17 Aug 2023, personal communication

55. Crockett, R.A., King, S.E., Marteau, T.M., et al., 'Nutritional labelling for healthier food or non-alcoholic drink purchasing and consumption', *Cochrane Database of Systematic Reviews* 2018;2:CD009315

56. Bleich, S.N., Wolfson, J.A., Jarlenski, M.P., 'Calorie changes in large chain restaurants: Declines in new menu items but room for improvement', *American Journal of Preventive Medicine* 2016;50:e1–e8

57. British Heart Foundation, 'Breakfast cereals ranked best to worst', https://www.bhf.org.uk/ informationsupport/heart-matters-magazine/nutrition/ breakfast-cereals-ranked-best-to-worst

58. Traversy, G., Chaput, J.P., 'Alcohol consumption and obesity: An update', *Current Obesity Reports* 2015;4:122–30

59. Robertson, T.M., Alzaabi, A.Z., Robertson, M.D., Fielding, B.A., 'Starchy carbohydrates in a healthy diet: The role of the humble potato', *Nutrients* 2018;10

60. USDA, 'Dietary Guidelines for Americans 2015–2020. Cut Down on Added Sugars', 2015 https://health.gov/sites/default/ files/2019-10/DGA_Cut-Down-On-Added-Sugars.pdf; National Health Service, 'The Eatwell guide', https://www. nhs.uk/live-well/eat-well/food-guidelines-and-food-labels/ the-eatwell-guide/

Chapter 12

1. World Health Organization, https://www.who.int/news-room/ fact-sheets/detail/obesity-and-overweight

2. Bray, G.A., Nielsen, S.J., Popkin, B.M., 'Consumption of high-fructose corn syrup in beverages may play a role in the epidemic of obesity', *American Journal of Clinical Nutrition* 2004;79:537–43

3. *Independent*, https://www.independent.co.uk/news/business/ news/britain-spending-more-on-eating-out-than-dining-at- home-412517.html

4. Statista, https://www.statista.com/statistics/239410/ us-food-service-and-drinking-place-sales/

5. Young, L.R., Nestle, M., 'The contribution of expanding portion sizes to the US obesity epidemic', *American Journal of Public Health* 2002;92:246–9; British Nutrition Foundation, 'Portion size: Cause and solution to overweight and obesity?', 2022 https://www.nutrition.org.uk/news/ portion-size-cause-and-solution-to-overweight-and-obesity/

6. BBC, http://news.bbc.co.uk/1/hi/education/7200949.stm

7. The Food Foundation, 'The Broken Plate 2022', report, 2022 https://foodfoundation.org.uk/press-release/ major-report-highlights-impact-britains-disastrous-food-policy

8. Ritchie, H., for Our World In Data, 'Three billion people cannot afford a healthy diet', 2021 https://ourworldindata.org/ diet-affordability

9. Hager, K., Du, M., Li, Z., et al., 'Impact of produce prescriptions on diet, food security, and cardiometabolic health outcomes: A multisite evaluation of 9 produce prescription programs in the United States', *Circulation: Cardiovascular Quality and Outcomes* 2023:e009520

10. Speakman, J.R., de Jong, J.M.A., Sinha, S., et al., 'Total daily energy expenditure has declined over the past three decades due to declining basal expenditure, not reduced activity expenditure', *Nature Metabolism* 2023;5:579–88

11. UK TV Licensing, https://www.tvlicensing.co.uk/about/media-centre/news/report-reveals-latest-uk-tv-watching-trends-NEWS35

12. Statista, https://www.statista.com/statistics/186833/average-television-use-per-person-in-the-us-since-2002/

13. Raynor, D.A., Phelan, S., Hill, J.O., Wing, R.R., 'Television viewing and long-term weight maintenance: Results from the National Weight Control Registry', *Obesity* 2006;14:1816–24

14. *Guardian*, https://www.theguardian.com/world/2021/jan/22/children-health-screen-times-covid-crisis-sleep-eyesight-problems-digital-devices

15. UK National Statistics, National Travel Survey, https://www.gov.uk/government/statistics/national-travel-survey-2021/national-travel-survey-2021-household-car-availability-and-trends-in-car-trips#:~:text=The%20proportion%20of%20households%20with%20one%20car%20was%2045%25%20in,)%20to%2022%25%20in%202021

16. Wikipedia, https://en.wikipedia.org/wiki/Car_ownership

17. Forbes Advisor, https://www.forbes.com/advisor/car-insurance/car-ownership-statistics/#:~:text=the%20data%20Embed-,How%20Many%20Americans%20Own%20a%20Car%3F,up%20from%2091.2%25%20in%202017

18. Livingtransport.com, https://www.livingtransport.com/results.php?t=asset&search=235

19. Save the Children, https://www.savethechildren.org.uk/news/media-centre/press-releases/children-today-62-percent-less-likely-to-play-outside-than-their#:~:text=Just%2027%25%20of%20children%20said,in%20just%20a%20few%20generations

20. Department for Transport, 'Walking and Cycling Statistics, England: 2019', 2020

21. Buehler, R., Pucher, J., Merom, D., Bauman, A., 'Active travel

in Germany and the U.S. Contributions of daily walking and cycling to physical activity', *American Journal of Preventive Medicine* 2011;41:241–50

22. Nuffield Trust, https://www.nuffieldtrust. org.uk/resource/obesity?gclid=CjwKCAjw-vmkBhBMEiwAlrMeFx1AEZQounGpHkLsabm0eOEHifQzE-hWPl8_Y6GiC1mhkZ1GHSMomRoCVo0QAvD_BwE; Statista, https://www.statista.com/forecasts/1166451/ overweight-population-share-forecast-in-the-united-states

23. Kim, Y., Je, Y., 'Dietary fiber intake and total mortality: A meta-analysis of prospective cohort studies', *American Journal of Epidemiology* 2014;180:565–73; Aune, D., Giovannucci, E., Boffetta, P., et al., 'Fruit and vegetable intake and the risk of cardiovascular disease, total cancer and all-cause mortality: A systematic review and dose-response meta-analysis of prospective studies, *International Journal of Epidemiology* 2017;46:1029–56; Schwingshackl, L., Schwedhelm, C., Hoffmann, G., et al., 'Food groups and risk of all-cause mortality: A systematic review and meta-analysis of prospective studies', *American Journal of Clinical Nutrition* 2017;105:1462–73; Eleftheriou, D., Benetou, V., Trichopoulou, A., La Vecchia, C., Bamia, C., 'Mediterranean diet and its components in relation to all-cause mortality: Meta-analysis', *British Journal of Nutrition* 2018;120:1081–97; Jayedi, A., Soltani, S., Abdolshahi, A., Shab-Bidar, S., 'Healthy and unhealthy dietary patterns and the risk of chronic disease: An umbrella review of meta-analyses of prospective cohort studies', *British Journal of Nutrition* 2020;124:1133–44; Zhang, Y.B., Pan, X.F., Chen, J., et al., 'Combined lifestyle factors, all-cause mortality and cardiovascular disease: A systematic review and meta-analysis of prospective cohort studies', *Journal of Epidemiology and Community Health* 2021;75:92–9

24. KevinMD.com, https://www.kevinmd.com/2023/04/why-weight-loss-drugs-are-not-the-answer-to-obesity.html

25. Thomson, A., 'Wonder drugs can't solve our obesity problem', *The Times*, 6 Sept 2023

26. Sylvester, R., '(Not so) big in Japan', *The Times: Magazine*, 21 Oct 2023

27. Sylvester, R., '(Not so) big in Japan', *The Times: Magazine*, 21 Oct 2023; Puska, P., Jaini, P., 'The North Karelia Project:

Prevention of cardiovascular disease in Finland through population-based lifestyle interventions', *American Journal of Lifestyle Medicine* 2020;14:495–9

28. Jousilahti, P., Laatikainen, T., Salomaa, V., Pietilä, A., Vartiainen, E., Puska, P., '40-Year CHD mortality trends and the role of risk factors in mortality decline: The North Karelia Project experience', *Global Heart* 2016;11:207–12

29. Thies, D.R., White, M., 'Is obesity policy in England fit for purpose? Analysis of government strategies and policies, 1992–2020', *The Milbank Quarterly* 2021;99:126–70

30. Metcalfe, S., Sasse, T., 'Tackling obesity: Improving policy making on food and health', Institute for Government, 2023

31. Blundell, J., 'Behaviour, energy balance, obesity and capitalism', *European Journal of Clinical Nutrition* 2018;72:1305–9

32. BBC, https://www.bbc.com/future/bespoke/made-on-earth/the-great-bicycle-boom-of-2020.html

33. *Guardian*, https://www.theguardian.com/society/2023/may/18/obese-patients-cost-nhs-twice-much-healthy-weight-study#:~:text=Obese%20patients%20with%20a%20BMI,save%20nearly%20%C2%A314bn%20annually

Appendix

1. UK Government, Regulation (EU) No 1169/2011 of the European Parliament and of the Council, 2011 https://www.legislation.gov.uk/eur/2011/1169/contents; UK Government, 'The Food Information Regulations 2014', 2014 https://www.legislation.gov.uk/uksi/2014/1855/made

2. US Food and Drug Administration, 'Food Labeling & Nutrition', 2023 https://www.fda.gov/food/food-labeling-nutrition

3. Sood, N., Baker, W.L., Coleman, C.I., 'Effect of glucomannan on plasma lipid and glucose concentrations, body weight, and blood pressure: Systematic review and meta-analysis', *American Journal of Clinical Nutrition* 2008;88:1167–75

4. Sherwood, T., for British Heart Foundation, 'We're all eating too much salt – here's why that matters', 2022 https://www.bhf.org.uk/what-we-do/news-from-the-bhf/news-archive/2022/march/why-matters-eat-too-much-salt

Index